Practice Tests, Questions and Answers for the **UKCAT**

Practice Tests, Questions and Answers for the **UKCAT**

Rosalie Hutton and Glenn Hutton

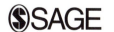

Los Angeles | London | New Delhi
Singapore | Washington DC

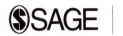

Learning Matters
An imprint of SAGE Publications Ltd
1 Oliver's Yard
55 City Road
London EC1Y 1SP

SAGE Publications Inc.
2455 Teller Road
Thousand Oaks, California 91320

SAGE Publications India Pvt Ltd
B 1/I 1 Mohan Cooperative Industrial Area
Mathura Road
New Delhi 110 044

SAGE Publications Asia-Pacific Pte Ltd
3 Church Street
#10-04 Samsung Hub
Singapore 049483

Editor: Amy Thornton
Development editor: Jennifer Clark
Production controller: Chris Marke
Project management: Deer Park Productions
Marketing manager: Catherine Slinn
Cover design: Toucan
Typeset by: Pantek Media
Printed by: MPG Books Group, Bodmin, Cornwall

FSC

First published 2010
Second edition published 2012

Library of Congress Control Number: 2012931686

British Library Cataloguing in Publication data

A catalogue record for this book is available from the
British Library

ISBN 978 0 85725 869 4
ISBN 978 0 85725 785 7 (pbk)

Contents

Dedication

To the memory of Jessie Mary Orme and Hazel Orme

Introduction

This book is a companion to *Passing the UKCAT and BMAT*. The original book, which is updated annually, is written essentially as a development tool. It contains detailed instructions on how to prepare for the UKCAT, analysis of the types of questions used in the Test, practice tests and worked examples. This book is for those people who have an understanding of the areas being tested and who wish to further develop their skills and exam technique. Although the use of textbooks can be no guarantee of passing an examination, it should develop your understanding and skills of the areas being tested and enable you to realise your full potential. Further, these tests will also identify any areas where you may still require some development.

In total, *Practice Tests, Questions and Answers for the UKCAT* provides over 500 questions across the five subtests. This is the second edition of the book and contains 25 per cent of new material across all of the subtests. Please note that questions and answers in relation to the BMAT are not included in this book.

Part I and Part II of the book each contain full tests comprising of: Verbal Reasoning, Quantitative Reasoning, Abstract Reasoning and Decision Analysis. The answers and rationale for each question are provided in Part IV of the book.

Part III of the book is dedicated to the Non-Cognitive Analysis subtest. This subtest basically measures an individual's personality in terms of their most likely traits. Currently, the results from this subtest are not used in the decision-making process, i.e. pass or fail, though this may change in the future. There are very few texts providing actual tests for this area, and this book replicates the subtest that candidates are likely to encounter. There are a total of 160 questions in this subtest. However, in 2011 the UKCAT Consortium decided that candidates would not be required to take the Non-Cognitive Analysis subtest (the behavioural test). The Consortium have stated on their website that this test'…will be reintroduced into future years of testing after further research has taken place on the use of these scores.' After much consideration it was determined to retain this particular test in the book because (a) it is not clear when it will be reintroduced; (b) it would still be of general interest to the reader who may be required to sit similar behavioural tests, for example, when seeking employment or during their working lives; and (c) this test is cross-referenced from *Passing the UKCAT and BMAT* book, which itself provides a brief overview of the test.

It is anticipated that you may wish to sit the tests simulating examination conditions, and instructions in relation to timing have been provided before each subtest. You will need a paper and pencil in order to write down the answers to the questions and for the Quantitative Reasoning subtest to undertake mathematical calculations.

Part I
Practice test 1

Chapter 1
Verbal Reasoning practice subtest 1

The Verbal Reasoning subtest is an on-screen test that consists of 44 items associated with 11 reading passages. For each reading passage there are four questions in the form of statements. Three answer options are provided for each statement: True; False; Can't Tell. Only one of these options is correct. A period of twenty-two minutes is allowed for the subtest, with one minute for instruction and the remaining twenty-one minutes for items.

The answers and rationale for this subtest can be found on page 123.

Passage I: discrimination and mental health

Social stigma and prejudice are examples of discrimination, and mental health service users can often find that society and the community are unwilling to engage with them. This can be expressed directly in the form of explicit rejection, ridicule or aggression, or indirectly in the form of dismissal or avoidance. This is largely based on fear and misunderstanding of what mental health means, and it is not uncommon for questions of capability and risk to be presented as reasons for exclusion. Indirect discrimination is often more complex to identify, as it results from a misunderstanding and adaptation rather than a direct and explicit rejection or exclusion. For those with mental health issues it is based more on attitudes and social norms. Some types of stigma and stereotyping can be defined as indirect discrimination, for example presuming that an individual is unable to make decisions or unable to take part in a cognitive activity.

Passage I: question 1
Discrimination affects the recipient's sense of self-worth and overall self-image.

A. True

B. False

C. Can't Tell ✓

Passage I: question 2

A lack of awareness can lead to people with mental health issues being excluded from society.

A. True

B. False

C. Can't Tell

Passage I: question 3

Rarely questions of capability and risk are presented as reasons for excluding those with mental health problems.

A. True ✗

B. False

C. Can't Tell

Passage I: question 4

Mental health creates a barrier to social interaction, services, employment and training.

A. True

B. False ✓

C. Can't Tell

Passage II: patient choice

If your GP refers you to a specialist you can choose the hospital you want to be treated at. You can choose any hospital in England that meets the NHS standards and this could include independent or private hospitals which are free as part of the Choice agenda. To support Choice, most GP practices use a national IT system called Choose and Book. You can choose the hospital with the best reputation, shortest waiting times, or simply the one that is most convenient. Choice of hospitals may not be appropriate for all services. Services where speedy access to diagnosis and treatment are particularly important are not required to offer a choice of hospital. This includes: emergency attendances or admissions, patients attending a Rapid Access Chest Pain Clinic under the two-week maximum waiting time, and patients attending cancer services under the two-week maximum waiting time. Mental health and maternity services are also not included, although your GP may offer you a choice of providers if you are referred for these services.

Passage II: question 5

Because of the Choice agenda you will always be able to choose the hospital which you want to be treated at except for mental health and maternity services.

A. True

B. False ✓

C. Can't Tell

Passage II: question 6

Patients suffering from cancer and chest pains do not have to be offered a choice of which hospital they can attend.

A. True ✓

B. False

C. Can't Tell

Passage II: question 7

GPs in Wales and Scotland do not have access to the Choose and Book IT system.

A. True

B. False ✓

C. Can't Tell

Passage II: question 8

Rapid Access Chest Pain Clinics and cancer services are not provided by independent and private hospitals.

A. True ✓

B. False

C. Can't Tell

Passage III: diabetes and sleeping disorders

According to the NHS, type 2 diabetes, which is often associated with obesity, affects about 2.3 million people in the UK, with at least 500,000 more who are not aware that they have the condition. Research has linked type 2 diabetes and sleeping disorders, suggesting there is a connection between diabetes and the way the body responds to the 24-hour cycle of light and dark. New genetic research points to a gene involved in detecting melatonin – a hormone that is part of the body's internal clock – and an increased risk of diabetes. The findings of the research will raise the possibility of genetic tests to identify people vulnerable to developing type 2 diabetes.

Passage III: question 9
People who are obese are more likely to suffer from sleeping disorders.

A. True

B. False

C. Can't Tell

Passage III: question 10
Genetic tests are available to identify people with type 2 diabetes.

A. True

B. False

C. Can't Tell

Passage III: question 11
There are about 2.8 million people in the UK affected by type 2 diabetes.

A. True

B. False   X

C. Can't Tell

Passage III: question 12
People with type 2 diabetes are often awake during the night and sleep during the day.

A. True

B. False

C. Can't Tell

Passage IV: cost of life-saving drugs reduced

A radical deal has been struck between drug companies and the Health Service for the cost of life-saving drugs to be significantly reduced. Currently, a number of effective drugs are not used because they are too expensive. Previously drug companies would charge what they believed the market would bear, but under the new agreement companies will offer flexible prices. They will still be able to charge what they want, say for new cancer or heart drugs, but companies will enter into negotiations with the Health Service for a realistic 'value' to be placed on the drug. The new scheme may see savings of about £200m, in the first year, rising to £300m in subsequent years.

Passage IV: question 13

In offering more flexible prices for their products the profits made by drug companies will decline.

A. True

B. False

C. Can't Tell

Passage IV: question 14

People are dying because the Health Service cannot afford to buy drugs that would keep them alive.

A. True

B. False

C. Can't Tell

Passage IV: question 15

The fact that drug companies are willing to enter into negotiations with the Health Service about drug pricing shows they are more concerned with people living and dying rather than profiting from the misfortune of others.

A. True

B. False   ̐

C. Can't Tell

Passage IV: question 16

When the Health Service can afford to buy more effective drugs the death rate in relation to people suffering heart disease and cancer will be significantly reduced.

A. True

B. False

C. Can't Tell

Passage V: cross-curriculum themed classes

In an overhaul of education for 5–11-year-olds it is proposed that history, geography and science will be removed from the curriculum and their content taught through cross-curriculum themed classes. It is considered that the teaching of rigid subject areas in primary schools was making children's knowledge and understanding shallow. In addition to the curriculum changes there is a proposal that teachers encourage children's social and emotional well-being in an explicit recognition that schools must help to cure some of the 'social ills' facing society.

Passage V: question 17
History, geography and science will no longer be taught in primary schools.

A. True

B. False

C. Can't Tell

Passage V: question 18
Teachers have a responsibility for the social fabric of society.

A. True

B. False

C. Can't Tell

Passage V: question 19
Children under 11 have only a superficial understanding of history, geography and science.

A. True

B. False

C. Can't Tell

Passage V: question 20
Cross-curriculum themed classes will result in primary school children having a better understanding of history, geography and science.

A. True

B. False

C. Can't Tell

Passage VI: educational success and communication skills

A think tank has reported that children growing up in the most deprived homes need to be taught to speak and have lessons in empathy and self-control. Some children from the most deprived homes have only been 'grunted' at by their parents, and empathy and self-control will not have been learnt at home. Communication skills are seen as the road to educational success, but in poorer homes children only hear 500 different words a day compared to 1,500 in a better-off household. From this it is estimated that about one in ten children start school unable to talk in sentences or understand simple instructions. In some parts of the country this can rise to 50% of four- and five-year-olds. It is believed parents in deprived areas often feel alienated from a child they did not want, may be depressed by their circumstances or not be functioning socially and emotionally because of drugs or alcohol.

Passage VI: question 21
Children from deprived homes will not attain the same educational standards as children from middle-class homes.

A. True

B. False

C. Can't Tell

Passage VI: question 22
In poorer homes less articulate conversations take place between carers and children.

A. True

B. False

C. Can't Tell

Passage VI: question 23
Parents who are drug addicts or alcoholics are more likely to have children who have difficulty communicating when they first attend school.

A. True

B. False

C. Can't Tell

Passage VI: question 24

In better-off households children are likely to hear five times as many different words spoken in the home each day as children from deprived homes.

A. True

B. False

C. Can't Tell

Passage VII: *patterns of communicable disease*

The patterns of communicable disease are the result of the interactions between the infectious agent, the host and the environment. The source of infection may be human, there may be animal reservoirs such as brucellosis in cattle or leptospirosis in rats, or reservoirs may exist in the environment in the water or soil. There are a number of modes of transmission between the source and the host through direct or indirect transmission (by vectors or vehicles). Vehicles such as water or food carry the infective agent while vectors such as mosquitoes for malaria are part of the life cycle. The transmission of infection may be by inhalation, ingestion, direct skin or mucosal contact, sexual contact, injection, or cross-placental routes. The susceptibility of the host is influenced by age, natural immunity, artificial immunity (active or passive), nutritional status and immune suppression.

Passage VII: question 25

Immunisation can protect people from contacting certain communicable diseases.

A. True

B. False

C. Can't Tell

Passage VII: question 26

Communicable diseases are continually changing and new communicable diseases emerging.

A. True

B. False

C. Can't Tell

Passage VII: question 27

A person's age, diet and lifestyle choices have little impact on their susceptibility to disease.

A. True

B. False

C. Can't Tell

Passage VII: question 28
The atmosphere is a vehicle that can carry an infective agent.

A. True

B. False

C. Can't Tell

Passage VIII: the meaning of 'normal'

Different people use the word 'normal' in different ways. A philosopher views the normal as the most usual. Psychologists and statisticians refer to normal as the middle range of a distribution of values (i.e. statistically normal). A sociologist defines 'normal' as that which is in line with a rule for a particular social or cultural group in society. The Oxford English Dictionary defines 'normal' as 'conforming to a standard'. In medicine 'normal' is often used to mean an absence of physiological pathology. In common speech, 'normal' may simply mean 'not abnormal, not strange'.

Passage VIII: question 29
'Normal' can refer to the lack of a significant deviation from the average.

A. True

B. False

C. Can't Tell

Passage VIII: question 30
Violating social norms or standards may be normal dependent on the social and cultural group to which a person belongs.

A. True

B. False

C. Can't Tell

Passage VIII: question 31

People are often referred to as 'strange' if they are seen not to agree with the views and principles of the majority.

A. True

B. False

C. Can't Tell

Passage VIII: question 32

In medicine, everyone who has a disease is considered to be 'abnormal'.

A. True

B. False

C. Can't Tell

Passage IX: Internet restrictions

A survey of managers aged 35 and under found that two-thirds of employers monitor staff use of the Internet during working hours and block access to sites deemed irrelevant to the job. This has been branded as 'old fashioned', with senior executives not encouraging the benefits of exploiting new technology. 16% of managers described their senior executives as dinosaurs. Senior executives were pessimistic that staff wanted access to the Internet for research, professional development and other aspects of getting the job done. 65% of organisations monitored Internet usage, and this rose to 88% in the police. Also, 65% blocked access to 'inappropriate' sites, with this rising to 89% in local government and 90% in the utilities.

Passage IX: question 33

There is a 'generation gap' in views about the use of Internet technology at work.

A. True

B. False

C. Can't Tell

Passage IX: question 34

Senior executives consider Internet usage as a waste of time.

A. True

B. False

C. Can't Tell

Passage IX: question 35
Monitoring Internet usage is higher in the police because of their accountability.

A. True

B. False

C. Can't Tell

Passage IX: question 36
35% of organisations do not block access to 'inappropriate' Internet sites.

A. True

B. False

C. Can't Tell

Passage X: Europe sets working week limit

The European Parliament has scrapped the special treatment granted to some sovereign states to allow people to work in excess of the 48 hours a week limit set by the European Union. However, the UK government intends to carry on the battle to retain the right to longer working hours, believing it gives a choice to UK workers to work in excess of 48 hours if they so wish. The trade unions are in favour of the European maximum 48-hour limit that is averaged out over a one-year period. The government believe the working hours limit would cost the UK economy tens of billions of pounds over the next 10 years. In addition to the 48 hour working week, the European Parliament has also decided that 'inactive' on-call time for employees, such as doctors, should be counted as working hours, a position the government considers will hamper the National Health Service.

Passage X: question 37
If the European Parliament decision is accepted by the UK no one will work more than 48 hours a week.

A. True

B. False

C. Can't Tell

Passage X: question 38
Because 'inactive' on-call time for doctors will be counted as working hours the National Health Service will need to recruit more doctors.

A. True

B. False

C. Can't Tell

Passage X: question 39

Trade unions are not in favour of their members working overtime.

A. True

B. False

C. Can't Tell

Passage X: question 40

People working in excess of the 48-hour working time limit make a significant contribution to the UK economy.

A. True

B. False

C. Can't Tell

Passage XI: new technology helps disabled

Access to education for people with disabilities and learning difficulties is now being helped by new technology. Sophisticated software now turns speech into written form for the hearing impaired, while printed words are transformed into sounds at the click of a button for the blind. Those suffering from dyslexia can alter the size or colour on a printed document to make it easier to read. The ability to make effective use of this new technology can depend on a student's age and IT literacy. This is particularly true of mature disabled students who did not grow up with new technology. However, the difficulties in accessing learning tend to lie not in the student's disability or learning problem, but in the task they are expected to perform where time may be a crucial factor. What can take an able-bodied person a few minutes can mean hours of work for someone with a disability. Overall disabled students have generally become agile users of new technologies, developing personal strategies depending on their needs and making full use of whatever technical support is on offer.

Passage XI: question 41

Technology is more of a benefit than a barrier to learning.

A. True

B. False

C. Can't Tell

Passage XI: question 42

Technology will help all people with disabilities and learning difficulties obtain academic qualifications.

A. True

B. False

C. Can't Tell

Passage XI: question 43

Universities have to offer all students equal learning opportunities.

A. True

B. False

C. Can't Tell

Passage XI: question 44

New technology allows students to study in previously unimagined ways.

A. True

B. False

C. Can't Tell

Chapter 2
Quantitative Reasoning practice subtest 1

The Quantitative Reasoning subtest consists of 36 items associated with tables, charts and/ or graphs. A period of twenty-three minutes is allowed for the test, with one minute for instruction and twenty-two minutes for items.

Remember that each of the questions is always accompanied by five possible answers, A, B, C, D and E, and that only ONE answer is correct. Also remember to read through all five competing answers before selecting what you consider to be the correct answer. By reading the four 'incorrect' answers you should confirm that your choice is in fact correct.

The answers and rationale for this subtest can be found on page 132.

Questions 1 to 4 relate to the table below. This provides the 'scores' of a sample of men and women who have sat the on-screen hazard simulation test as part of the driving licence test requirement. The test has a maximum possible score of 70 and the pass mark is a minimum 37 correct responses.

Respondent	Score	Respondent	Score
1 (Female)	38	11 (Male)	40
2 (Male)	29	12 (Female)	57
3 (Female)	47	13 (Female)	39
4 (Female)	39	14 (Female)	35
5 (Male)	44	15 (Female)	46
6 (Male)	23	16 (Male)	33
7 (Male)	37	17 (Female)	31
8 (Male)	43	18 (Male)	37
9 (Female)	54	19 (Female)	45
10 (Male)	36	20 (Female)	41

1. What is the percentage of the sample who successfully passed the on-screen hazard simulation test?

    A. 50%

    B. 55%

    C. 60%

    D. 65%

    E. 70%

2. What is the mode of the females' scores who sat the on-screen hazard simulation test?

    A. 31

    B. 39

    C. 41

    D. 46

    E. 57

3. What is the range of the males' scores who sat the on-screen hazard simulation test?

    A. 21

    B. 23

    C. 33

    D. 39

    E. 44

4. In relation to the scores for the on-screen hazard simulation test, which one of the following statements is correct?

    A. More than half of the respondents scored above the mean.

    B. The ratio of males that passed the test compared to the number of successful females was 1:3.

    C. Less than half of the respondents scored above the mean.

    D. More than half of the male respondents attained a score above the mean.

    E. Less than half of the female respondents attained a score above the mean.

Questions 5 to 8 relate to a medium-sized enterprise whose products are mainly for markets outside the European Union (EU). The table below provides a list of the current postal charges to non-EU countries.

SURFACE MAIL				AIRMAIL		
weight	letters	packets		weight	letters	packets
not over	price	price		not over	price	price
				10g	£6.60	£7.45
20g	58p	99p		20g	£6.60	£7.45
60g	£1.00	99p		60g	£7.25	£7.45
100g	£1.41	99p		100g	£7.86	£7.45
150g	£1.99	£1.32		140g	£8.51	£7.76
500g	£5.86	£3.65		180g	£9.16	£8.10
750g	£8.62	£5.32		220g	£9.74	£8.42
1000g	£11.36	£6.98		240g	£10.04	£8.57
1500g	£16.87	£10.31		280g	£10.61	£8.89
2000g	£21.64	£13.22		300g	£10.91	£9.06

Surface Mail: letters over 2000g cannot be sent by surface mail, packets over 2000g, for each 50g thereafter add 28p

Airmail: letters/packets over 300g, for every 20g up to 500g add 16p, every 20g up to 1kg add 20p, and every 200g above 1kg add 18p

5. The company has four letters each weighing 150g and five packets, three of which weigh 200g and the remainder each weigh 300g. As a percentage, how much cheaper would surface mail be compared to airmail?

A. 30.6%

B. 32.5%

C. 57.8%

D. 67.5%

E. 74.2%

6. Unlike surface mail, airmail rates are currently subject to VAT at 20%. If VAT were not charged on airmail rates, what would be the cost of sending 25 letters each weighing 100g?

    A. £158.20

    B. £164.10

    C. £170.20

    D. £180.80

    E. £191.48

7. Which one of the following statements is correct?

    A. Airmail letters weighing 1 kilogram cost an extra £6.60 in addition to the price of a 300g letter.

    B. Compared to airmail it is cheaper to send a packet weighing 2.5kg by surface mail.

    C. It is always cheaper to send packets by airmail compared to letters by airmail.

    D. Sending a 100g letter by surface mail is about $\frac{1}{10}$ of the price of sending a 100g letter by airmail.

    E. The cost of sending a 4 kilogram packet by surface mail would be £32.84.

8. The company secretary has 27 letters to post with each letter being of the same weight. The total weight of the letters is 4.5 kilograms. What would be the cost of surface mail for 27 letters?

    A. £53.73

    B. £79.60

    C. £117.20

    D. £146.50

    E. £158.22

Questions 9 to 12 are about a town bookshop, and shown in the table below are some of the broad classifications used by the bookshop in cataloguing their books and the number of books in stock per classification.

Book Classifications	Current Stock Level
Paperback Fiction	12,750
Biography	3,800
History	5,700
Science	3,450
Geography	2,275
Medical	3,500
Nature	4,125
Education	7,600
Reference	10,300
Ancient World	1,900

9. To the nearest whole number, what percentage of stock in the bookshop is classified as 'history'?

    A. 3%

    B. 5%

    C. 7%

    D. 10%

    E. 12%

10. The total selling price of the paperback fiction books currently in stock is £101,362.50. How much is the actual selling price, per paperback fiction book, where there is a promotion of 4 for the price of 3 on all paperback fiction books?

    A. £4.46

    B. £5.16

    C. £5.96

    D. £6.17

    E. £6.45

11. The total selling price of the medical books currently in stock is £31,324.00. If the bookshop buys the medical books for $\frac{2}{3}$ of the selling price how much profit would it make if $\frac{3}{8}$ of the current stock were sold (to 2 decimal places)?

    A. £1,305.17

    B. £1,976.43

    C. £2,610.34

    D. £3,915.50

    E. £10,441.33

12. What is the range of the number of books currently in stock in the bookshop by classification?

    A. 2,450

    B. 5,150

    C. 7,050

    D. 9,250

    E. 10,850

Questions 13 to 16 relate to the information contained in the pie chart below. This information shows the average number of text messages per person per month, for last year, across ten countries. The percentage change over the past five years for each country is shown in parentheses.

Average monthly text messages per person (IDATA)

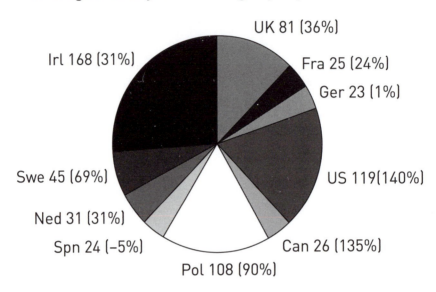

13. From the information contained in the pie chart which one of the following statements is correct?

   A. The number of countries in which people average more than 80 text messages a month exceeds those with less than this number.

   B. Countries whose average number of text messages per person per month is less than 25 account for one tenth of those included in the survey.

   C. The average number of texts per person for Ireland (Irl) is 2,016 per annum, up from 128 per month five years ago.

   D. The average percentage change over the past five years for the top five countries where people send the most text messages per month is less than 70%.

   E. Spn (Spain) has the lowest average number of text messages per person per month.

14. What percentage of countries has an average number of text messages in excess of 32 per person per month?

   A.   25%

   B.   30%

   C.   40%

   D.   50%

   E.   60%

15. What is the ratio of the number of messages per person per month in the UK and US combined compared to the total number of messages per person per month living in the other countries within the survey?

   A.   1:3

   B.   1:6

   C.   2:7

   D.   3:8

   E.   4:9

16. The average cost of a text message for all countries is £0.05p. How much would the annual average number of text messages per individual cost in Ireland (€1 = £0.80p) and the US ($1 = £0.68p)?

   A.   €10.50 and $88.00

   B.   €76.80 and $57.40

   C.   €100.80 and $71.40

   D.   €126.00 and $105.00

   E.   €226.80 and $177.40

Questions 17 to 20 relate to the figure which shows the birth rates in Scotland over a 4-year period according to the age range of the women who gave birth, shown as a percentage of the total births.

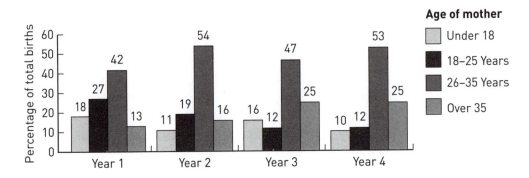

17. Which one of the following statements is supported by the information in the figure above?

   A. Between Year 1 and Year 4 the birth rate for women over 35 was about a third more than for women under 18.

   B. Between Year 1 and Year 4 the birth rate for women aged 26–35 remained within a margin of 12%.

   C. Between Year 1 and Year 4 the birth rate for women under 18 decreased by nearly three-quarters.

   D. Between Year 1 and Year 4 the average percentage birth rate for women aged 18–25 years was over 20%.

   E. Between Year 1 and Year 4 the percentage of births for women aged over 35 increased by less than half.

18. If 750 women aged 26–35 gave birth to one child each in Year 2, how many women aged 18–25, to the nearest 50, gave birth in the same year, assuming that they each had one child?

   A. 350

   B. 300

   C. 250

   D. 200

   E. 150

19. Which one of the following statements is supported by the information in the figure above?

A. Over the 4 years the percentage birth rate for women aged 26–35 was consistently three times greater than for the other age ranges of women added together.

B. The least significant rise or fall in birth rates over 4 years was in relation to women aged 26–35 years.

C. The lowest percentage swing in birth rates over the 4 years was in relation to women aged over 35.

D. The single highest fall in birth rates during the 4 years was in relation to women aged 18–25.

E. Between Year 3 and Year 4 women aged over 35 were twice as likely to give birth than women under the age of 18.

20. What is the average percentage of total births to women aged over 35, between Year 1 and Year 4?

Closest to

A. 25%

B. 20%

C. 15%

D. 12%

E. 10%

Questions 21 to 24 are about the table below. This shows the results of a survey about the weights of 120 people, 24 to 32 years of age, selected at random to participate in a study on obesity.

Weight in kilograms (kg)	<50	51–60	61–70	71–80	81–90	>90
Number of people	10	20	21	29	26	14

21. How many people weigh less than 71 kilograms?

    A. 10

    B. 20

    C. 41

    D. 51

    E. 81

22. What can you say categorically about the weight of 25% of the people surveyed?

    A. They are less than 70 kilograms.

    B. They are more than 70 kilograms and less than 90 kilograms.

    C. They are at most 60 kilograms.

    D. They are less than 80 kilograms.

    E. They are at least 71 kilograms.

23. What fraction of the people surveyed weigh in excess of 80 kilograms?

    A. $\dfrac{3}{8}$

    B. $\dfrac{1}{3}$

    C. $\dfrac{1}{4}$

    D. $\dfrac{1}{2}$

    E. $\dfrac{3}{4}$

24. What is the ratio of the number of people who weigh less than 61 kilograms compared to the number who weigh 61 kilograms and above?

    A. 1:3

    B. 1:4

    C. 2:3

    D. 3:4

    E. 3:5

Questions 25 to 28 are about a college and the student population. The college currently has 19,876 students registered and 8,241 of these are studying a science subject. Also 6,037 of the students are part-time. It is not possible to study a science subject part-time.

25. Approximately, what is the percentage of students who are part-time?

   A.   7%

   B.   15%

   C.   20%

   D.   25%

   E.   30%

26. What is the approximate ratio of students studying science compared to the rest of students at the college?

   A.   2:3

   B.   2:5

   C.   3:2

   D.   3:4

   E.   3:5

27. Student loans are not available to part-time students and those studying science subjects obtain grants and do not need to obtain a student loan. If all of those students entitled to a student loan actually obtain a loan, how much is the total cost, to the nearest £m, of providing the loans if each student is in receipt of £2,300?

   A.   £13m

   B.   £14m

   C.   £19m

   D.   £32m

   E.   £46m

28. The student accommodation for the college is divided into blocks. 21 blocks can hold 48 students in each, whilst 38 blocks can hold 93 students in each. What is the best approximation for the maximum capacity of students in the college accommodation blocks?

    A.   1,000

    B.   2,000

    C.   3,500

    D.   4,600

    E.   6,000

Questions 29 to 32 relate to a floor layer who is tiling the floor of five bathrooms in a small hotel before the bathroom furniture is installed. Four of the five bathrooms are of the same dimensions as shown in the figure below. The fifth bathroom is, in area, $\frac{3}{4}$ the size of one of the other bathrooms.

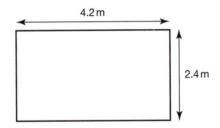

29. What is the total area of flooring that requires tiling to the nearest whole metre?

    A.   40m²

    B.   44m²

    C.   48m²

    D.   52m²

    E.   56m²

30. The tiles that are being used measure 30cm². How many tiles, to the nearest whole tile, would be required for one of the larger bathrooms?

    A.   82

    B.   88

    C.   92

    D.   96

    E.   112

Before laying the tiles the hotel owner decides to fit showers in the four larger bathrooms as shown in the diagram below. The floor area to be tiled has been reduced by the size of the shower. Note the measurements are now in millimetres.

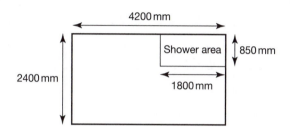

31. In order to find the new floor area of the bathroom that requires tiling, which one of the following is correct?

    A. $(4200 \times 2400) - (1800 \times 850)$

    B. $(2400 - 850) + (4200 - 1800)$

    C. $(4200 \times 1800) - (2400 - 850)$

    D. $((2400 - 850) + (4200 - 1800)$

    E. $(850 + 2400) - (4200 \times 2400)$

32. The floor layer has estimated that he will need about 500 tiles to complete the job. At the builders' merchants the tiles cost £2.75 each but there is a discount of 12% per hundred. Also there is a buy-back policy of £1.25 per tile. If the builder uses 430 tiles, how much will he have paid if he returns the unused tiles?

    A. £1,035.50

    B. £1,080.00

    C. £1,122.50

    D. £1,210.00

    E. £1,375.00

Questions 33 to 36 relate to the table below that provides information on strikes and stoppages in the United Kingdom over a 12-month period.

Strikes and stoppages in the UK: 12-month period

Number of disputes	Reasons for disputes	Working days lost
52	pay	48,300
12	pattern of hours	6,580
24	redundancy	26,125
5	union matters	2,460
11	working conditions	4,900
25	manning/work allocation	18,260
25	dismissal/discipline	8,700

33. What is the mean of the number of disputes over the 12-month period?

   A. 12

   B. 22

   C. 24

   D. 25

   E. 27

34 What is the mode of the number of disputes over the 12-month period?

   A. 17

   B. 21

   C. 25

   D. 28

   E. 32

35. What is the range of the total working days lost over the 12-month period?

   A. 8,700

   B. 16,475

   C. 25,425

   D. 36,690

   E. 45,840

36. In relation to the table which one of the following statements is correct?

   A. On average, redundancy had more days lost than any other reason for disputes.

   B. The average number of working days lost in relation to disputes over pay is less than those in relation to union matters.

   C. The lowest number of disputes accounted for the least number of working days lost.

   D. Manning/work allocation and dismissal/discipline disputes together accounted for over half of the total number of working days lost.

   E. Compared to pay, the number of pattern of hours disputes were about 10% less.

Chapter 3
Abstract Reasoning practice subtest 1

The Abstract Reasoning subtest is an on-screen test that consists of 65 items associated with 13 pairs of Set A and Set B shapes. Five test shapes are presented with each pair of Set A and Set B shapes and there are three answer options for each test shape: Set A, Set B or Neither Set. Only ONE of the three answer options is correct. Each test shape is presented with the pair of Set A and Set B shapes on a separate screen with the three answer options below. A period of sixteen minutes is allowed for the test, with one minute for instruction and the remaining fifteen minutes for items.

The answers and rationale for this subtest can be found on page 139.

Questions 1 to 5

Set A

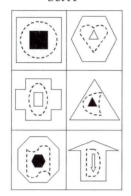

Set B

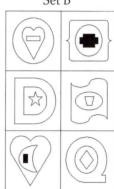

Test shapes

Question 1	Question 2	Question 3	Question 4	Question 5

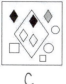
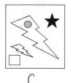
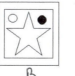
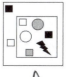

B   C   A   B   C

Questions 6 to 10

Set A

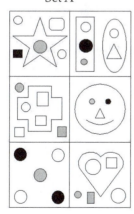

Set B

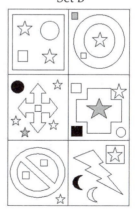

Test shapes

Question 6	Question 7	Question 8	Question 9	Question 10

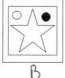

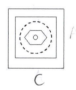

C   C   B   A   B

Questions 11 to 15

Set A

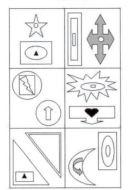

Set B

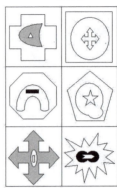

Test shapes

| Question 11 | Question 12 | Question 13 | Question 14 | Question 15 |

B

A

C

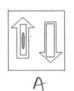

A

C

Questions 16 to 20

Set A

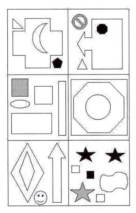

Set B

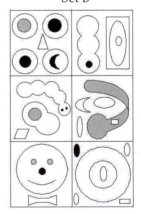

Test shapes

| Question 16 | Question 17 | Question 18 | Question 19 | Question 20 |

B

B

Questions 21 to 25

Set A

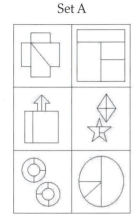

Set B

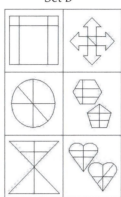

Test shapes

| Question 21 | Question 22 | Question 23 | Question 24 | Question 25 |

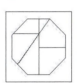

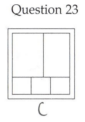

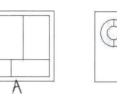

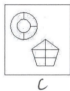

A

B

C

A

C

Questions 26 to 30

Set A

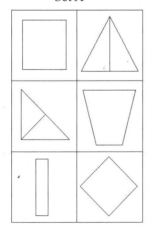

Set B

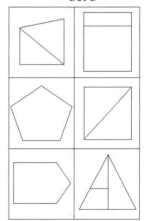

Test shapes

| Question 26 | Question 27 | Question 28 | Question 29 | Question 30 |

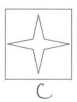

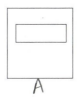

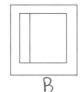

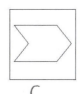

C

A

B

C

A

Questions 31 to 35

Set A

Set B

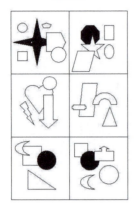

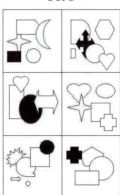

Test shapes

| Question 31 | Question 32 | Question 33 | Question 34 | Question 35 |

Questions 36 to 40

Set A

Set B

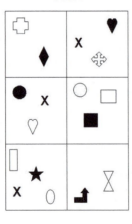

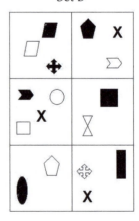

Test shapes

| Question 36 | Question 37 | Question 38 | Question 39 | Question 40 |

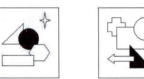 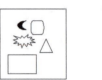

Questions 41 to 45

Set A

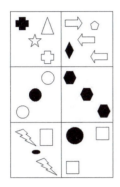

Set B

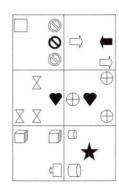

Test shapes

Question 41 Question 42 Question 43 Question 44 Question 45

Questions 46 to 50

Set A

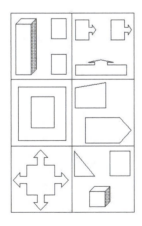

Set B

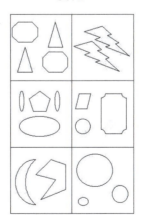

Test shapes

Question 46 Question 47 Question 48 Question 49 Question 50

Questions 51 to 55

Set A

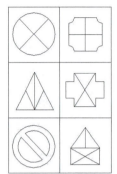

Set B

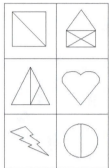

Test shapes

Question 51	Question 52	Question 53	Question 54	Question 55
				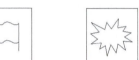

Questions 56 to 60

Set A

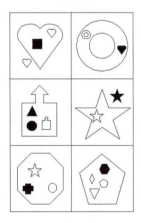

Set B

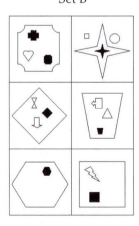

Test shapes

Question 56	Question 57	Question 58	Question 59	Question 60

Questions 61 to 65

<table>
<tr><td align="center">Set A</td><td align="center">Set B</td></tr>
</table>

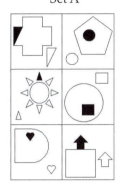 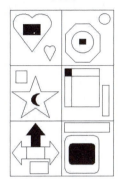

Test shapes

Question 61	Question 62	Question 63	Question 64	Question 65

Chapter 4
Decision Analysis practice subtest 1

The Decision Analysis subtest is an on-screen test that consists of one scenario and 26 associated items. The scenario may contain text, tables and other types of information. The 26 items have four or five response options and for some items more than one of the options may be correct. Where more than one of the response options is correct this is clearly identified within the item. A period of thirty minutes is allowed for the test, with one minute for instruction and the remaining twenty-nine minutes for items.

The answers and rationale for this subtest can be found on page 146.

The Buzzards and the Kites

The Buzzards and the Kites are a group of ten children who regularly play together. They communicate with each other by using codes so that other children or adults cannot spoil their fun and games (of course their parents have access to the codes). The Buzzards and the Kites would like to increase their group to twelve and they are going to select the two children who can grasp their codes in the quickest time by decoding 26 messages. To pass this test you will be required to interpret the coded questions and select the best option or options from those listed. The information from the codes may not always be complete and may be in any order, but you are asked to make your 'best judgement' based on this information and not on what you might consider to be reasonable.

Table: the Buzzards and the Kites codes

Action codes	People codes	Toy codes	Time codes	Like codes
A = run	☺ = me	⮷ = bike	🍽 = dinner	11 = happy
B = walk	⛊ = them	⛵ = boat	☽ = night	22 = sad
C = jump	♀ = mother	🚗 = car	♈ = lunch	33 = cry
D = fly	♂ = father	📄 = book	bb = breakfast	44 = laugh
E = fall	Ⓟ = police	✎ = crayon	ww = weekend	55 = jealous
F = ride	☻ = enemies	▯ = bucket	hh = holiday	66 = greedy
G = fight	101 = us	➤ = Frisbee	nn = now	77 = tall
H = climb	202 = we	& = scooter	tt = tomorrow	88 = small
I = opposite	303 = you	? = skipping rope	yy = yesterday	99 = smile
J = negative	404 = brother		cc = year	00 = angry
K = increase	505 = sister	# = paint	am = morning	
L = play	606 = cousin	∧ = kite	pm = afternoon	
M = combine	707 = neighbour	} = skateboard		
⌁ = swim	808 = doctor	▸▸ = spade		
⛴ = sail		◎ = ball		
✊ = talk				
⌇ = sleep				

Question 1

What is the best interpretation of the following coded message:
👜K, 📑K, 404, (11 99), ☺

A. Sailing makes my brother happy.

B. Books on sailing please my brother.

C. My brother is pleased when I give him a book.

D. Books on sailing make my brother smile.

E. My brother gave me a book on sailing.

Question 2

What is the best interpretation of the following coded message:
(404 606), 404, 606, G, FK, &K, ☺

A. My brother and cousin fight over scooters.

B. Scooters are the cause of arguments in our family.

C. My brother and cousin argue when riding their scooters.

D. My cousin and brother ride their scooters together.

E. My family argue over who will ride the scooter.

Question 3

What is the best interpretation of the following coded message:
(505 }), ☺, A, (Ⓟ 🚗)

A. My sister skateboarded into the police car.

B. The police car is faster than my sister's skateboard.

C. The police told my sister not to skateboard near cars.

D. The police car ran over my sister's skateboard.

E. My sister left her skateboard and ran to the police car.

Question 4

What is the best interpretation of the following coded message:
(am pm), L, ☺ ♦♦♦ , (J bb ⊤ ♦○♦)

A. We play all day and forget to eat.

B. We play after breakfast, lunch and dinner.

C. Eating gets in the way of play.

D. When we play in the morning we forget breakfast.

E. We are always ready for our meals when we play all day.

Question 5

What is the best interpretation of the following coded message:
🚲K, 101, &K, 101, AK (NB: **Two** options are correct.)

A. Their bikes are faster than our scooters.

B. Our bikes are faster than our scooters.

C. Our scooters aren't as fast as our bikes.

D. Our scooters aren't as fast as their bikes.

E. Our bikes and scooters are both fast.

Question 6

What is the best interpretation of the following coded message:
🚲K, hh, ⚓K, 11, ☺, M 505 ♦ ⊤ 404

A. My family swim and cycle on holiday.

B. Swimming and cycling is enjoyed by all of us.

C. Family holidays involve swimming and cycling.

D. Holidays are more enjoyable if you swim and cycle.

E. My family enjoy swimming and cycling on holiday.

Question 7

What is the best interpretation of the following coded message:

707, ♠, ✹, 808

A. Our neighbour telephoned mum about the doctor.

B. Mum telephoned the doctor for the lady next door.

C. Mum said the neighbour called the doctor.

D. The doctor is mum's neighbour.

E. The lady next door to mum is a doctor.

Question 8

What is the best interpretation of the following coded message:
👽 I, 202, ♠, 11, 101, Υ, M(202 👽 I)

A. Mum is not happy if we have lunch with our enemies.

B. We are happy that mum lets us have lunch together.

C. Our friends are happy when mum lets us have lunch together.

D. Our friends like it when we ask them to lunch.

E. Our enemies are not happy when we have lunch with mum.

Question 9

What is the best interpretation of the following coded message:

}, 202, ♟♟♟, 707, 00

A. We were angry and took the neighbour's skateboard.

B. Our neighbour was angry and took their skateboard.

C. Their neighbour was angry and took their skateboard.

D. We were angry that the neighbour took our skateboard.

E. Our neighbour does not like us skateboarding.

Question 10

What is the best interpretation of the following coded message:
33 K, 77 I, 505, E, &, ☺

A. My big sister fell off her scooter and cried.

B. I cried when my sister fell off her scooter.

C. My small sister is always falling off her scooter.

D. My sister and me often fall off the scooter.

E. My small sister fell off her scooter and cried.

Question 11

What is the best interpretation of the following coded message:

🚗 K, 202, J ➷, ☽

A. We had to sleep in the car last night.

B. The cars did not keep us awake last night.

C. The cars kept us awake.

D. We had no sleep last night due to traffic.

E. Traffic is noisy at night outside our bedroom.

Question 12

What is the best interpretation of the following coded message:

🏊 , 202, 101, 🗑 K, hh, ⏩ K

A. We swim and play with our buckets and spades on holiday.

B. We take our buckets and spades on holiday.

C. We play with our buckets in the water on holiday.

D. Our holidays are spent on the beach with buckets and spades.

E. We either swim or play with our buckets and spades.

Question 13

What is the best interpretation of the following coded message:
Ⓟ , ♂ , C K, Ƴ, F

A. After lunch the policeman went for a bike ride.

B. The policeman skipped lunch and rode off on his bike.

C. The policeman jumped onto the bike and rode off for lunch.

D. Police cyclists take their lunch with them.

E. The policeman said he would jump on his bike and come over.

Question 14

What is the best interpretation of the following coded message:
M(404 505), ⚲, ☺, ☺, M(K 22 33 00), G (NB: **Two** options are correct.)

A. Mum gets very emotional when my siblings and I argue.

B. Mum cries and gets angry when I fight with my brother.

C. Mother is angry when I make my brother and sister cry.

D. My siblings make me angry when they upset mum.

E. When I fall out with my siblings mother gets really upset.

Question 15

Which **two** of the following would be the most useful additions to the codes when attempting to convey the following message:

My family are flying off for a holiday in the sun later this year.

A. plane

B. hot

C. cold

D. time

E. airport

Question 16

What is the best interpretation of the following coded message:

L, tt, 202, ♔♔♔ , ♣ː, ☺, M(⚲ ⚊ 🚗 ⚊ } ◎)

A. I spoke to my friends to see whether we are playing tomorrow.

B. I chat with my friends about which toys we will play with tomorrow.

C. Tomorrow we are going bike riding, skateboarding and playing ball.

D. It is up to my friends which toys we will play with tomorrow.

E. My friends and I will discuss what we are playing tomorrow.

Question 17

What would be the best way to encode the following message:

My family smile and laugh a lot because we are very happy.

A. ☺ , M(404 ♟ 505 ♈), 202, 99, 44, K 11

B. K(99 44), 202, K 11, ☺, M(404 ♟ 505 ♈)

C. ☺ , M(404 ♟ 505 ♈), K(99 33), 101, K 11

D. K(99 44), 202, 11, ☺, (404 ♟ 505 ♈)

E. 202, ☺, K(99 44), M(404 ♟ 505 ♈)

Question 18

What is the best interpretation of the following coded message:

♟, ♈, 707, 🍽, I 66, ♣ː

A. Mum and dad say the neighbour gives generous dinner portions.

B. Mum and dad have invited the greedy neighbour to dinner.

C. The neighbour says that mum and dad are greedy.

D. Mum and dad asked the neighbour to dinner.

E. The neighbour generously asked mum and dad to dinner.

Question 19

What is the best interpretation of the following coded message:

E, 88 **?**, 101, I 🚢 , ⬓

A. We sailed the boat tied to the rope.

B. The skipping rope made our boat sink.

C. The rope fell off and our boat sank.

D. The boat sank so we played with the skipping rope.

E. Our boat sailed with the small rope attached.

Question 20

What is the best interpretation of the following coded message:
K D, ^, L, 202, nn ww, I, M(☺ 👫)

A. This weekend we are having a kite flying game against each other.

B. We are going to play kite flying this weekend.

C. I will not oppose my friends in the weekend kite flying contest.

D. This weekend's kite flying is for my friends and me only.

E. I will fly my kite opposite my friends this weekend.

Question 21

Which **two** of the following would be the most useful additions to the codes when attempting to convey the following message:

The police said that the paint poured on our car was criminal damage.

A. break

B. throw

C. drop

D. harass

E. crook

Question 22

What is the best interpretation of the following coded message:

M(bb ⍦ 🍽), 202, hh, M(⍦ ⍦ ☺ 404 505)

A. We eat our meals with mum and dad when on holiday.

B. I have breakfast, lunch and dinner with my family.

C. We have breakfast, lunch and dinner together on holiday.

D. We have all our meals together when on holiday.

E. We just have our main meal together when on holiday.

Question 23

What is the best interpretation of the following coded message:
#, E, 88 🗑 , 88 707

A. The child from next door fell over the tin of paint.

B. The neighbour's tin of paint fell over.

C. The bucket of paint fell on the neighbour.

D. The tin of paint fell on the child.

E. The neighbour fell on the bucket of paint.

Question 24

What is the best interpretation of the following coded message:
K M(A C H B ⚓), 202, L, M(⍦ ⍦ ☺ 404 505 606)

A. Our family swim, walk, run and climb together.

B. We all play together.

C. Our family have very active hobbies.

D. Mother and father like us all to be very active.

E. Very active play is good for us all.

Question 25

What would be the best way to encode the following message:

The doctor had to fight to stop my sister from drowning.

A. J ⚓ , H, 808, ☺ , 505, I B

B. G, 808, ☺ , 505, I B, J ⚓

C. 808, ☺ , 505, I B, J ⚓ , D

D. ⚓ , H, 808, ☺ , 505, I B

E. G, 808, ☺ , 404, I B, J ⚓

Question 26

What is the best interpretation of the following coded message:
✏, Υ , #, nn, 🚗 , 55

A. The neighbour is jealous of dad's new car.

B. The paint colour of dad's new car is green.

C. Father had to have the car painted.

D. Dad was jealous and wanted a new car.

E. Now dad has changed the car for a green one.

Part II
Practice test 2

Chapter 5
Verbal Reasoning practice subtest 2

The Verbal Reasoning subtest is an on-screen test that consists of 44 items associated with 11 reading passages. For each reading passage there are four questions in the form of statements. Three answer options are provided for each statement: True, False or Can't Tell. Only one of these options is correct. A period of twenty-two minutes is allowed for the subtest, with one minute for instruction and the remaining twenty-one minutes for items.

The answers and rationale for this subtest can be found on page 153.

Passage I: MRSA and *Clostridium difficile*

After a surprise inspection by the Healthcare Commission revealed dirty bedpans and concerns about the adequacy of training for staff, a big London hospital has been warned that it must raise hygiene standards. The hospital has a good record on MRSA and *Clostridium difficile*, the two most rampant hospital superbugs, but the Commission says its systems are not sound enough to prevent a potentially serious hygiene lapse. Inspectors found bedpans and commodes that had been cleaned but were visibly dirty and marked as being ready for use. In the endoscopy suite it was not clear whether flexible tubes that are inserted into the body for diagnosis and treatment were ready for sterilisation or had already been decontaminated, even though this had previously been brought to the hospital's attention. An audit by the hospital's own trust also found that only 6 out of 10 staff were washing their hands properly, but the trust's board was not informed. The board had also been informed that attendance for mandatory infection control training by staff was acceptable, but in fact it was low. Only three out of nine hygiene audits planned for the previous 12 months had been carried out. These breaches of the Government's hygiene code gave the Commission cause for concern, in spite of the low incidence of infections. The hospital reported 22 cases in *C. difficile* between April and June.

Passage I: question 1
The Healthcare Commission is responsible for hygiene inspections of National Health Service and trust hospitals.

A. True

B. False

C. Can't Tell

Passage I: question 2

One of the major issues at the hospital inspected appears to be a lack of communication between the staff and the trust board.

A. True

B. False

C. Can't Tell

Passage I: question 3

Twenty-two cases of *Clostridium difficile* at the hospital in a three-month period is considered particularly high.

A. True

B. False

C. Can't Tell

Passage I: question 4

This is not the first inspection of the hospital by inspectors from the Healthcare Commission.

A. True

B. False

C. Can't Tell

Passage II: cultural identity

We all have a cultural identity and shared outlook which provides us with a sense of 'belonging'. This belonging may be to a small group, such as a university sports team, or a large group, such as a nation or religion. Within those groups we have shared prejudices about other teams, other nations and other religions. A confrontation or even an interaction with another group, or culture, can be threatening because it implies a difference of opinion with different answers to fundamental questions of why we live the way we do. Culture shock is a phrase used to describe our reaction when we encounter behaviour that we would not necessarily consider appropriate even if it is the norm in another culture. A common reaction to different cultures is fear, which can lead to distrust and hostility.

Passage II: question 5

It is often a natural reaction for a person to be prejudiced when encountering other cultures.

A. True

B. False

C. Can't Tell

Passage II: question 6

All wars can be traced back to fundamental cultural differences.

A. True

B. False

C. Can't Tell

Passage II: question 7

In a multicultural society such as Britain there is a greater acceptance and tolerance of differing religious beliefs than is the case in other countries.

A. True

B. False

C. Can't Tell

Passage II: question 8

The membership of both small and large social groups encourages a competitive and even prejudicial outlook in relation to other such social groups.

A. True

B. False

C. Can't Tell

Passage III: jet aircraft biofuels

Air travel generates 3 per cent of global carbon dioxide emissions. It is one of the fastest rising contributors to climate change, but the search for a greener alternative to kerosene jet fuel has been problematic. Airlines cannot use standard first-generation biofuels such as ethanol because these would freeze at high altitude. In addition, environmentalists argue that manufacturing biofuels can produce more emissions than they absorb when growing, and can also displace agricultural crops and push up the price of food. However, the search for an environmentally friendly fuel for aeroplanes is moving forward. The world's first flight powered by a second-generation biofuel, derived from plants that do not compete with food crops, has recently taken place in New Zealand. An Air New Zealand jumbo jet with a 50–50 mix of jet fuel and oil from jatropha trees in one of its four engines successfully undertook a two-hour test flight, without the need for any modification of the engines. The biofuel was made from jatropha nuts, which are up to 40% oil, harvested from trees grown on marginal land in India, Mozambique, Malawi and Tanzania. An American airline is shortly to run a test flight that will use a mixture of jatropha-derived biofuel and fuel made from algae in one of its engines. Again, algae are not a food source and can be grown in arid regions and virtually anywhere. However, Greenpeace has warned against over-interpreting the results from the test flights. They believe it will not mean an end to the use of kerosene jet engines, as the amount of jatropha that would be needed to power the entire aviation section can never be produced in a sustainable way.

Passage III: question 9
The oils from jatropha nuts and algae are the preferred oils for use with kerosene jet fuel.

A. True

B. False

C. Can't Tell

Passage III: question 10
It is likely that eventually the use of kerosene jet engines will be a thing of the past.

A. True

B. False

C. Can't Tell

Passage III: question 11
Algae and the jatropha trees can be grown in the arid regions of the world and virtually anywhere.

A. True

B. False

C. Can't Tell

Passage III: question 12

The use of biofuels is of particular concern to environmentalists because of the increase in emissions caused by growing crops specifically for biofuel use.

A. True

B. False

C. Can't Tell

Passage IV: universities defy government cap

Universities have accepted 35,000 more students than in the previous year despite a government cap of 13,000. This capping followed the finding that there was a £200 million black hole in their university financing. The government are intending to fine universities for every student admitted over the official limit, which could cost universities millions of pounds. There were an additional 60,000 applications for places in the current year, comprising a 10 per cent increase in students overall but a 19.5 per cent rise among students over 25 years of age. The universities themselves believe that to some extent the anxieties in the media about the government capping could have exacerbated the natural urge for students to sort out their applications. University applications for the following year are already up 14 per cent on the previous year with the number of applications standing at 150,000. There are also record numbers of non-EU students opting to study in the UK, the number of overseas students doubling in the past 10 years. Fees for non-EU students are not regulated and they are now the biggest source of income for universities after the government.

Passage IV: question 13

A large number of suitably qualified students were not prevented from starting a degree due to universities defying an order to restrict the number of places.

A. True

B. False

C. Can't Tell

Passage IV: question 14

The number of over-25s successfully applying for university places now exceeds the number of under-25s.

A. True

B. False

C. Can't Tell

Passage IV: question 15

The rise in the number of mature students enrolling at universities has been prompted by the over-25s being made, or being at risk of being made redundant and job insecurity.

A. True

B. False

C. Can't Tell

Passage IV: question 16

Universities welcome non-EU students to apply for places in order to provide much needed income.

A. True

B. False

C. Can't Tell

Passage V: speed limiters

A transport advisory body has recommended that speed limiters should be fitted to cars and lorries to reduce carbon emissions and cut accidents. The Commission for Integrated Transport and the Motorists' Forum claim that accidents involving injuries could be cut by 12 per cent if the system were adopted universally – with a manual override system – and by more if the speed limiter was mandatory and always on. Speed limiters would use satellite navigation technology to read the road's speed limit and adjust the vehicle's accelerator. Using the system on urban roads with a 30mph limit could increase fuel consumption and emissions, because cars operate more efficiently above that speed. However, there should be significant reductions on roads where the limit is 70mph. It is recommended that in the first instance speed limiters should be fitted to vehicles for newly qualified drivers and those convicted of dangerous driving. However, some people believe that the use of speed limiters could have dangerous consequences and could make road safety worse. For example, drivers may not be able to accelerate out of dangerous situations. Also there is an understandable deep-rooted concern about Big Brother!

Passage V: question 17

Cars and lorries operate more efficiently between 30 and 70mph.

A. True

B. False

C. Can't Tell

Passage V: question 18
The introduction of speed limiters might lead to a greater infringement of civil liberties.

A. True

B. False

C. Can't Tell

Passage V: question 19
The impact in relation to lorries would be minimal as engines on lorries are already fitted with a speed limiter.

A. True

B. False

C. Can't Tell

Passage V: question 20
Fitting speed limiters to the vehicles of newly qualified drivers would not see a reduction in the number of accidents involving injuries.

A. True

B. False

C. Can't Tell

Passage VI: excessive alcohol

Research has shown that high alcohol intake can affect mental abilities and damage someone's ability to pay attention, remember things and make good judgements. Heavy drinkers are already known to be at increased risk of having an accident, being involved in violence and engaging in unprotected sex, but research identifying permanent brain damage is a new phenomenon. The research indicated that in the UK 23 per cent of men and 15 per cent of women drink more than twice the government's recommended daily limit. It also showed that people who have a few heavy drinking sessions undergo subtle brain changes making it harder to learn from mistakes and new ways of tackling problems because their brain function has been impaired. Alcohol-related brain damage is an increasing burden on the NHS, and patients who do not die early with the condition need long-term care costing £1,000 a week for the rest of their lives.

Passage VI: question 21

23 per cent of men and 15 per cent of women are running the risk of suffering permanent brain damage from excessive alcohol consumption.

A.   True

B.   False

C.   Can't Tell

Passage VI: question 22

People who have unprotected sex are more likely to drink excessive amounts of alcohol.

A.   True

B.   False

C.   Can't Tell

Passage VI: question 23

The majority of people with alcohol-related brain damage have a shorter life expectancy.

A.   True

B.   False

C.   Can't Tell

Passage VI: question 24

Men are twice as likely as women to be heavy drinkers.

A.   True

B.   False

C.   Can't Tell

Passage VII: influences on health

The normal internal environment (body status) is called homeostasis. The homeostatic reserve of the very young and very old is less than that of those in early and middle adult life; for example, there are more frequent occurrences of delirium with infection at the extremes of the age spectrum. Early upbringing will also influence health in later life. There are the possible positive and negative effects of childhood diet and exercise, parental smoking and alcohol use, and good and bad parenting. Many elderly people with multiple pathologies still consider themselves to be normal and healthy by virtue of the fact they can go about their day-to-day lives. Generally, older people see their health as functioning even in the presence of chronic disease while young people see health more as fitness.

Passage VII: question 25

People who have had bad parents are more at risk of chronic disease later in their lives.

A. True

B. False

C. Can't Tell

Passage VII: question 26

Those in middle adult life are less likely to suffer delirium with infection than old people.

A. True

B. False

C. Can't Tell

Passage VII: question 27

Parental smoking or alcohol abuse has no adverse effect on the health of their children's health in later life.

A. True

B. False

C. Can't Tell

Passage VII: question 28

Generally, older people are less concerned about their levels of fitness than simply being able to function in their daily lives.

A. True

B. False

C. Can't Tell

Passage VIII: community service

People who have been convicted of a criminal offence in England and Wales and sentenced to community service are now required to wear bright orange bibs when undertaking their community work. These controversial bibs are designed as public reminders that offenders cleaning graffiti or laying pavements are being punished and not paid. Some people have suggested that the scheme is medieval and not dissimilar to putting offenders in stocks; that it is about shaming people. However, the government consider that any shame felt by offenders is the shame and humiliation of having committed an offence and the resulting criminal record. They believe the public want to see that justice is being done, that community punishments are seen as effective and tough, and that such sentences may result in fewer people being sent to prison. However, the Probation Service has highlighted the fact that there have been a number of attacks on offenders undertaking community service and that the use of bright orange bibs is almost certain to increase the risk.

Passage VIII: question 29

The orange bib scheme will mean that fewer offenders will be sentenced to terms of imprisonment.

A. True

B. False

C. Can't Tell

Passage VIII: question 30

Those offenders who are sentenced to community service are ashamed at having committed and been convicted of a criminal offence.

A. True

B. False

C. Can't Tell

Passage VIII: question 31

Offenders who don't wear orange bibs when undertaking community service are less likely to be attacked than those wearing orange bibs.

A. True

B. False

C. Can't Tell

Passage VIII: question 32

People were put in stocks in medieval times to be shamed for their wrongdoing.

A. True

B. False

C. Can't Tell

Passage IX: cow tax

Green Party activists are pressuring the government to introduce a 'cow tax' to penalise farmers for owning belching and flatulent cattle and pigs. They consider this an environmental issue and say that farmers should be charged for rising levels of methane and other polluting nitrous gases emitted by farm animals. It is calculated that a farm with 30 dairy cows, 40 beef cattle or 200 pigs emits more than 100 tons of carbon equivalent each year. The 'cow tax' would demand a fee of about £100 for each cow and £20 for each pig. The farming lobby is up in arms about such a tax and believes even moderate size farms could see tax bills in thousands of pounds. This could put many farmers out of business, with a knock-on effect of wide-scale closures of food outlets across the country.

Passage IX: question 33

If the 'cow tax' were introduced farms with 200 pigs would see a reduction in the current 100 tons of carbon equivalent produced each year.

A. True

B. False

C. Can't Tell

Passage IX: question 34

If farms closed as a result of the 'cow tax' there would be a shortage in the supply of cattle and pig products.

A. True

B. False

C. Can't Tell

Passage IX: question 35

The emission of methane and other nitrous gases from cattle and pigs is considered a real environmental issue.

A. True

B. False

C. Can't Tell

Passage IX: question 36
Farm animals' belching and flatulence have a significant carbon footprint.

A. True

B. False

C. Can't Tell

Passage X: offenders' benefit claims

Two years after being released from prison, 47 per cent of offenders were on out-of-work benefits. During the two-year period overall, 75 per cent of offenders made a new claim to an out-of-work benefit at some point. On average, offenders leaving prison spent 48 per cent of the next two years on out-of-work benefits. 11 per cent of offenders released from prison are back in prison two years after being released. During the two-year period overall nearly half (46 per cent) of offenders started another prison sentence at some point. Offenders discharged from custody who claimed Job Seeker's Allowance (JSA) within 13 weeks of release spent 57 per cent of the next three years on out-of-work benefits, compared with 42 per cent for the average JSA claimant.

Passage X: question 37
Within two years of being released from custody 46 per cent of offenders started another prison sentence.

A. True

B. False

C. Can't Tell

Passage X: question 38
Non-offenders in receipt of Job Seeker's Allowance accounted for 42 per cent of all claimants.

A. True

B. False

C. Can't Tell

Passage X: question 39
89 per cent of offenders released from prison commit no further offences within two years of their release.

A. True

B. False

C. Can't Tell

Passage X: question 40

Offenders leaving prison spent on average 47 per cent of the next two years on out-of-work benefits.

A. True

B. False

C. Can't Tell

Passage XI: *fuel poverty*

Data from a recent survey indicates that 4.0 million households in England were classified as being in fuel poverty (18% of all households). This is three times the number of households that were in fuel poverty six years ago. As might be expected, the vast majority of people who have both low incomes and live in very energy-inefficient housing are in fuel poverty. Less obviously, two of the low-income groups with high rates of fuel poverty are single-person households of working age and those who live in rural areas. This is notable because these two groups have not been the focus of the last government's more general anti-poverty strategy. Households are considered by the Government to be in 'fuel poverty' if they would have to spend more than 10% of their household income on fuel to keep their home in a 'satisfactory' condition. It is thus a measure which compares income with what the fuel costs 'should be' rather than what they actually are. Whether a household is in fuel poverty or not is determined by the interaction of a number of factors, but the three obvious ones are: the cost of energy, the energy efficiency of the property and household income. The focus of government's more general anti-poverty strategy has tended to focus on children, older people and deprived urban areas.

Passage XI: question 41

Loft insulation and double-glazing have a considerable impact on the energy efficiency of a house.

A. True

B. False

C. Can't Tell

Passage XI: question 42

'Fuel poverty' is a measure that compares household income with the actual costs of fuel.

A. True

B. False

C. Can't Tell

Passage XI: question 43

People who live in rural communities are more likely to be classified as being in fuel poverty compared to people living in urban areas.

A. True

B. False

C. Can't Tell

Passage XI: question 44

'Fuel poverty' disproportionately affects single-person households of working age who are on low incomes.

A. True

B. False

C. Can't Tell

Chapter 6
Quantitative Reasoning practice subtest 2

The Quantitative Reasoning subtest consists of 36 items associated with tables, charts and/or graphs. A period of twenty-three minutes is allowed for the test, with one minute for instruction and the remaining twenty-two minutes for items.

Remember that each of the questions is always accompanied by five possible answers, A, B, C, D and E, and that only ONE answer is correct. Also remember to read through all five competing answers before selecting what you consider to be the correct answer. By reading the four 'incorrect' answers you should confirm that your choice is in fact correct.

The answers and rationale for this subtest can be found on page 162.

Questions 1 to 4 are about a registered charity that offers services and activities to adults with learning disabilities. The table below shows the activities on offer, the session length, the individual's cost per session, and the actual cost to the charity.

Activity	Time	User cost	Charity cost
Theatre company	6 hours	£37.50	£25.75
Art and crafts	4 hours	£15.00	£9.75
Wednesday life-links	6 hours	£12.00	£8.40
Friday life-links	6 hours	£12.00	£8.40
Shop training	6 hours	£32.50	£23.25
Rural crafts	3 hours	£7.75	£4.00
Weaving to work	2 hours	£2.50	£1.75
Yoga	1 hour	£4.00	£2.85
Football	2 hours	£2.00	£1.45
Badminton	1 hour	£2.50	£1.65
Sewing	2 hours	£2.50	£1.65
Discotheque	3 hours	£3.00	£2.00

1. The charity is offering a reduction of 15% for service users who book a block of twelve sessions with the theatre company. What would be the total cost to the user for these twelve sessions?

   A. £318.75

   B. £351.05

   C. £382.50

   D. £405.00

   E. £450.00

2. What is the range of user costs for all activities?

   A. £6.88

   B. £8.40

   C. £11.10

   D. £24.00

   E. £35.50

3. The charity cost relates to the cost of running the activity. The 'profit' made between the user cost and charity cost covers central overhead costs. In relation to shop training, what percentage of the user cost covers the central overheads?

   A. 18%

   B. 21%

   C. 25%

   D. 28%

   E. 32%

4. One of the service users has a personal budget of £78.20 per week. Their preferences are to attend the theatre company for one day, two sessions of rural craft, one session of badminton and one session of yoga. How much more money would they need if they also wanted to do one-day shop training?

   A. £9.45

   B. £13.80

   C. £18.70

   D. £21.55

   E. £25.10

Questions 5 to 8 relate to the table below that shows the top ten results of a half marathon (13 miles) for the categories of men and women. The time is shown in hours and minutes.

MEN	Time	WOMEN	Time
A Taylor	2.35	C Akabusi	2.49
F Simkins	2.36	A Bakewell	2.51
L Glossop	2.40	Y Jeavons	2.52
B Smith	2.41	P Karlson	2.58
M Khan	2.42	T Zukova	3.01
C Denston	2.46	S Pearson	3.02
K Verma	2.48	D Pearson	3.02
J Yani	2.48	B Collins	3.07
T Price	2.50	P Johnson	3.09
K Benson	2.52	D Fellows	3.10

5. What is the mean running time, in minutes, for the top ten women runners in the half marathon?

    A.   86.10 minutes.

    B.   128.40 minutes.

    C.   180.10 minutes.

    D.   188.40 minutes.

    E.   240.10 minutes.

6. What is the difference in minutes between the mode running times for the men's and women's half marathon?

    A.   14 minutes.

    B.   17 minutes.

    C.   21 minutes.

    D.   28 minutes.

    E.   35 minutes.

7. What is the median running time, in hours and minutes, for the top ten men runners in the half marathon?

    A.   2 hours 42 minutes.

    B.   2 hours 44 minutes.

    C.   2 hours 45 minutes.

    D.   2 hours 46 minutes.

    E.   2 hours 48 minutes.

8.   The half marathon event was recognised by the Amateur Athletics Association as a qualifying event for the forthcoming regional championships. The time required to qualify for the championships was under 2 hours 46 minutes for men and under 3 hours 5 minutes for women. What percentage of the men and women runners in the top ten obtained the qualifying time?

    A.   35%

    B.   40%

    C.   45%

    D.   50%

    E.   55%

Questions 9 to 12 refer to the pie chart below which groups the level of turnover of a number of professional rugby league clubs included in a 'UK Sport for All' survey. The number of rugby league clubs per group is shown in parentheses.

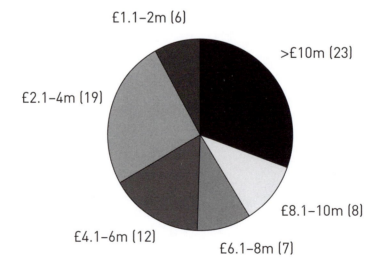

£1.1–2m (6)

>£10m (23)

£2.1–4m (19)

£8.1–10m (8)

£4.1–6m (12)

£6.1–8m (7)

9. What percentage, rounded to the nearest whole number, of rugby league clubs has a turnover in excess of £8m?

  A. 30%

  B. 37%

  C. 41%

  D. 45%

  E. 50%

10. 'UK Sport for All' wish to publish the results of the survey in Australia because of their close ties with rugby league and want the figures shown in Australian dollars. If £1 = A$2.10, what would be the minimum turnover in Australian dollars for those organisations with a turnover of £4.1–6m, to the nearest A$500,000?

  A. A$8,000,000

  B. A$8,500,000

  C. A$9,000,000

  D. A$9,500,000

  E. A$13,000,000

11. The rugby league clubs comprising this survey employ a total of 900 people, of whom 60% are employed by those clubs with a turnover in excess of £8m. The remaining employees are spread pro rata across the other clubs. How many employees, to the nearest round number, work for each rugby league club with a turnover of £2.1m to £4m?

  A. 8

  B. 10

  C. 12

  D. 15

  E. 21

12. What is the ratio of the number of rugby league clubs with a turnover of £6.1m to £10m compared to the rest of the rugby league clubs?

  A. 1:2

  B. 1:3

C. 2:3

D. 1:4

E. 1:5

Questions 13 to 16 are about the job of a painter and decorator who has been given the job of redecorating a lounge. The lounge is 7.5 metres long, 3.5 metres wide and 2.75 metres high and is shown in the diagram below.

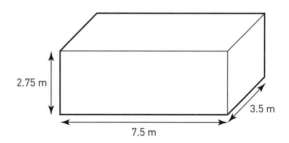

13. The owner of the property where the lounge is being redecorated wants the two long walls and one side wall painted in arctic white emulsion. A five-litre tin of arctic white emulsion costs £9.75 and will apply one coat to an area of 12 square metres. What is the total cost of paint required to apply two coats of paint, taking into account any excess paint?

    A. £29.25

    B. £36.55

    C. £48.75

    D. £87.75

    E. £107.25

14. The side wall that is not painted needs to be wallpapered using woodchip paper. One roll of wallpaper is 55 centimetres wide and 5 metres long. How many rolls of wallpaper will the decorator need, rounded up to the nearest whole number?

    A. 3

    B. 4

    C. 5

    D. 6

    E. 7

15. Before the decorator starts wallpapering, the owner decides he wants to fit a door in the side wall to lead out into a conservatory he is having built and also wallpaper the other side wall which has just been painted. The dimensions of the door are detailed in the drawing below:

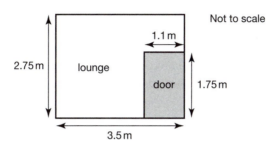

Assuming the wallpaper is 55cm wide, what is the total length of wallpaper in metres the decorator needs to wallpaper the two side walls?

A. 12m

B. 15m

C. 19m

D. 27m

E. 35m

16. Before painting and papering the lounge the decorator has estimated the cost of the job including his hourly rate. He has calculated that he will need about seven 5-litre tins of emulsion paint and no more than eight rolls of woodchip wallpaper. The paint normally costs £9.75 per tin but he gets it at trade with a 15% discount per tin. The woodchip wallpaper is £2.65 a roll with a same discount as the paint. He believes the job will take him 20 hours to complete and his labour charges are £18.50 an hour plus VAT at 20%. What is the total estimated cost for this job to the nearest £10.00?

A. £600.00

B. £575.00

C. £550.00

D. £520.00

E. £510.00

Questions 17 to 20 relate to an extract from an article on how crimes are being dealt with.

'More than 207,500 spot fines for disorder were issued last year, alongside 104,000 cannabis warnings and 362,900 police cautions. The increase means that for only the second time more crime was dealt with through summary justice than through the courts. The figures show that only 49% of 1.37m crimes detected last year resulted in a charge or court summons.'

17. Last year how many more people were dealt with by spot fines for disorder, cannabis warnings or police cautions than were dealt with by a charge or court summons?

   A. 24,300

   B. 14,900

   C. 7,450

   D. 3,100

   E. 2,800

18. In relation to all crime detected last year, what percentage of crime (to two decimal places) was dealt with by spot fines for disorder?

   A. 7.59%

   B. 15.15%

   C. 20.28%

   D. 26.50%

   E. 30.34%

19. What was the approximate ratio of cannabis warnings compared to police cautions?

   A. 1:5

   B. 2:3

   C. 2:7

   D. 2:9

   E. 3:5

20. In 10 years from these figures being published, detected crimes are forecast to increase by 18% when, if current trends continue, only 40% of these detected crimes will result in a charge or court summons. If this were the case what would be the number of police cautions in 10 years' time assuming they rise proportionately to spot fines and warnings, to the nearest whole number?

    A. 503,797

    B. 593,870

    C. 674,400

    D. 737,200

    E. 969,960

Questions 21 to 24 are about 'stopovers' and associated flying times (in hours) when travelling by air from the UK to Australia and New Zealand. These are presented in the table below.

Country	Local Time	UK to Stopover	Stopover to Australia	Stopover to New Zealand
Bali	GMT +8	16 hours 9,700 miles	$5\frac{1}{2}$ hours 2,800 miles	8 hours 4,125 miles
Dubai	GMT +4	$7\frac{1}{2}$ hours 3,750 miles	14 hours 7,300 miles	$18\frac{1}{2}$ hours 11,300 miles
Hawaii	GMT −10	17 hours 10,500 miles	10 hours 5,300 miles	$9\frac{1}{4}$ hours 4,900 miles
Fiji	GMT +12	23 hours 12,800 miles	$4\frac{1}{2}$ hours 2,300 miles	3 hours 1,500 miles
China	GMT +8	$11\frac{1}{4}$ hours 6,250 miles	$10\frac{3}{4}$ hours 5,650 miles	16 hours 9,750 miles

21. From the UK how much longer in hours does it take to get to New Zealand if you include a stopover in China of 4 days, than it does to get to Australia including a stopover in Dubai of 3½ days?

    A. 17¾ hours

    B. 18¼ hours

    C. 20¾ hours

    D. 24¼ hours

    E. 25¾ hours

22. The cost of a single business class fare from the UK to China has been calculated at £0.15 per mile, with the mileage from China to New Zealand calculated at an additional £0.05 per mile. The cost of a return fare is 15 per cent less than the total cost of a two-way individual single fare. From UK to China is 6,250 miles, and from China to New Zealand is 9,750 miles. What is the cost of the return fare to New Zealand via China?

    A.   £2,310.00

    B.   £3,176.25

    C.   £4,052.50

    D.   £4,908.75

    E.   £5,775.00

23. Two flights leave the UK on Monday at 10.00 hours, one bound for Dubai and one for Hawaii. The Dubai flight is adversely affected by inclement weather conditions and arrives at its destination 1 hour and 12 minutes behind schedule. The flight to Hawaii develops technical problems and is forced to land at New York JFK. It is grounded for 5 hours and 20 minutes before continuing on to Hawaii without any further disruption. What is the difference in local time between the two planes landing at their destination?

    A.   2 minutes

    B.   2 hours 58 minutes

    C.   4 hours 2 minutes

    D.   8 hours 58 minutes

    E.   12 hours 2 minutes

24. The airlines using the routes to Australia and New Zealand mainly use the Boeing 757 aircraft that has an average cruising speed of 550mph. The airlines are now looking at taking into service a new aeroplane, the Boeing 787 that has an average cruising speed of 570mph. When the 787 is taken into service what will be the flight duration for an aircraft travelling to Australia with a stopover at Fiji to the nearest ½ hour?

    A.   25 hours

    B.   25½ hours

    C.   26 hours

    D.   26½ hours

    E.   27 hours

Questions 25 to 28 relate to the population figures of the United Kingdom for the 20th century as shown in table below.

UK population (thousands) 1901 to 2001

	United Kingdom	England & Wales	Scotland	Northern Ireland
1901	38,328	32,612	4,479	1,237
1911	42,138	36,136	4,751	1,251
1921	44,072	37,932	4,882	1,258
1931	46,074	39,988	4,843	1,243
1941	48,216	41,748	5,160	1,308
1951	50,290	43,815	5,102	1,373
1961	52,807	46,196	5,184	1,427
1971	55,928	49,152	5,236	1,540
1981	56,352	49,634	5,180	1,538
1991	57,808	51,099	5,107	1,601
2001	59,009	52,211	5,123	1,675

25. If the population of the United Kingdom continues to grow at the rate it did between 1981 and 2001, what would be the projected population (thousands) in 2021?

   A.   60,984

   B.   61,782

   C.   62,237

   D.   62,808

   E.   63,115

26. Which one of the following statements is correct?

   A.   Between 1901 and 1911 the growth rate of the UK population averaged 5% per annum.

   B.   The 20th century saw the population of Northern Ireland increase by over half a million.

   C.   The populations of England and Wales, Scotland and Northern Ireland have all grown at a similar rate.

D. In the 20th century the percentage growth rate in Northern Ireland exceeded that in Scotland.

E. The population in England and Wales increased by almost 50% over the 20th century.

27. Expressed as a fraction, approximately what was the population of Scotland compared to that of England and Wales in 1941?

A. $\frac{1}{2}$

B. $\frac{1}{3}$

C. $\frac{1}{4}$

D. $\frac{1}{6}$

E. $\frac{1}{8}$

28. The UK population is growing older. In 1951 the proportion of the population over 50 was about 25% and by 1991 it was about 31%. Assuming a similar increase to the 1951 and 1991 figures, how many people (thousands) would be over 50 by 2001?

A. 18,708

B. 18,992

C. 19,178

D. 19,709

E. 21,833

Questions 29 to 32 are about Reginald Smythe who has entered the biannual Laconda Touring Rally driving his vintage Laconda motor vehicle from London to Le Mans in France.

29. The first stage of the rally is from London to Dover, a distance of 70 miles. Smythe drives the first 20 miles at an average speed of 30 mph, the next 40 miles at an average of 60 mph and the last 10 miles at an average of 30 mph. How long did it take Smythe to drive from London to Dover?

A. 1 hour 35 minutes

B. 1 hour 40 minutes

C. 1 hour 45 minutes

D. 1 hour 50 minutes

E. 1 hour 55 minutes

30. Shortly after leaving the ferry in Calais, Smythe joins the E1 motorway in the direction of Paris. After three hours he pulls into a service area. For the first ¼ of this journey he travels at a steady 90 kilometres per hour (kph) and for the remainder of the journey travels at 120 kph. How far has Smythe travelled in miles (to 2 decimal places) between Calais and the service area? (1 mile = 1.6 kilometres).

A. 170.67 miles

B. 192.35 miles

C. 210.94 miles

D. 277.27 miles

E. 337.50 miles

31. Before leaving Calais, Smythe filled his car with 75 litres of petrol as the petrol gauge was on empty. By the time he reached Le Mans Smythe estimated that the car had a third of a tank of petrol remaining even though he stopped to fill it up with another 75 litres at Rouen. Smythe estimates his car does 5.75 kilometres per litre of petrol. How many kilometres has Smythe travelled between Calais and Le Mans?

A. 575 kilometres

B. 628.75 kilometres

C. 668.25 kilometres

D. 718.75 kilometres

E. 862.50 kilometres

32. Smythe is allowed to drive his Lagonda round the Le Mans racing circuit, which measures 5 miles for one lap. In driving round the circuit Smythe drives at 80 mph for 3 minutes, 110 mph for 12 minutes and 140 mph for 15 minutes. How many full laps of the Le Mans circuit does Smythe complete?

A. 6 laps

B. 8 laps

C. 10 laps

D. 12 laps

E. 14 laps

Questions 33 to 36 relate to the figure below which shows the number of deaths in a county over four 5-year periods according to the age range of the people who have died, shown as a percentage of the total deaths.

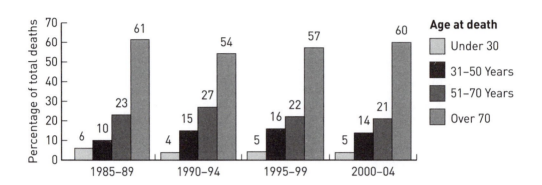

33. 575 women aged over 70 died between 1995 and 1999, accounting for $\frac{1}{3}$ of all deaths of people over 70. How many men aged over 70 died in the same period?

   A.   385

   B.   775

   C.   950

   D.   1,050

   E.   1,150

34. Which one of the following statements is supported by the information in the figure above?

   A.   Between 1985 and 2004 the average death rate for people over 70 exceeded the average death rate for people aged 31–50 by over 44%.

   B.   Between 1985 and 2004 the death rate for people aged 51–70 remained within a margin of 5%.

   C.   Between 1985 and 2004 the average percentage death rate for people 31–50 was in excess of 15%.

   D.   Between 1985 and 2004 the death rate for people under 30 remained constantly under 5% of the total number of deaths.

E. Between 1990 and 2004 the death rate for people aged 51–70 decreased by over three quarters.

35. Between 2000 and 2004 what is the approximate ratio of deaths of the over-70s compared to the 31–50-year-olds?

A. 2:5

B. 1:3

C. 3:1

D. 4:1

E. 5:2

36. Which one of the following statements is supported by the information in the figure above?

A. The percentage death rate for people aged 51–70 increased over the last two 5-year periods.

B. The largest percentage change in the death rate has occurred in people aged over 70.

C. The largest percentage change in the death rate for people aged 51–70 exceeded that of people aged 31–50.

D. The largest percentage change in the death rate has occurred in people aged 51–70.

E. The percentage change in the death rate for people aged under 30 remained constant.

Chapter 7
Abstract Reasoning practice subtest 2

The Abstract Reasoning subtest is an on-screen test that consists of 65 items associated with 13 pairs of Set A and Set B shapes. Five test shapes are presented with each pair of Set A and Set B shapes and there are three answer options for each test shape: Set A, Set B or Neither Set. Only ONE of the three answer options is correct. Each test shape is presented with the pair of Set A and Set B shapes on a separate screen with the three answer options below. A period of sixteen minutes is allowed for the test, with one minute for instruction and the remaining fifteen minutes for items.

The answers and rationale for this subtest can be found on page 171.

Questions 1 to 5

Set A

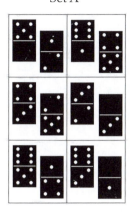

Set B

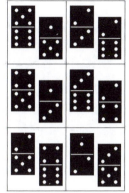

Test shapes

Question 1	Question 2	Question 3	Question 4	Question 5

 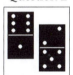

Questions 6 to 10

Set A

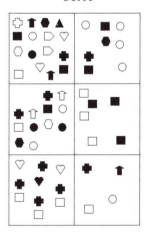

Set B

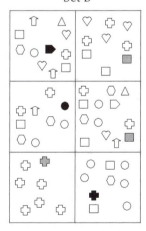

Test shapes

Question 6	Question 7	Question 8	Question 9	Question 10

 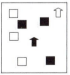 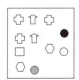 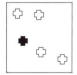

Questions 11 to 15

Set A

Set B

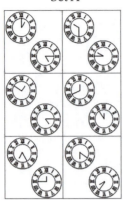

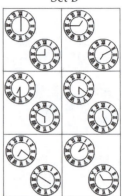

Test shapes

| Question 11 | Question 12 | Question 13 | Question 14 | Question 15 |

   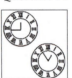

Questions 16 to 20

Set A

Set B

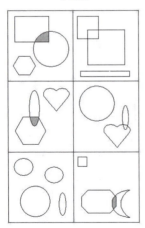

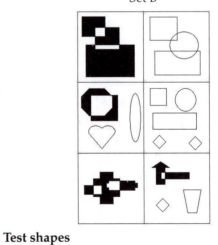

Test shapes

| Question 16 | Question 17 | Question 18 | Question 19 | Question 20 |

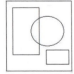 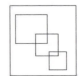 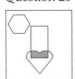

Questions 21 to 25

Set A

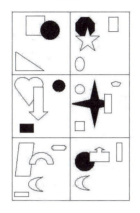

Set B

Test shapes

Question 21   Question 22   Question 23   Question 24   Question 25

Questions 26 to 30

Set A

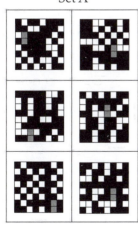

Set B

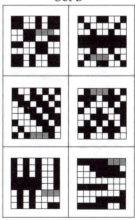

Test shapes

Question 26   Question 27   Question 28   Question 29   Question 30

   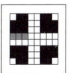

Questions 31 to 35

Set A

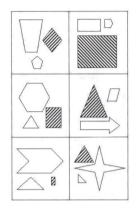

Set B

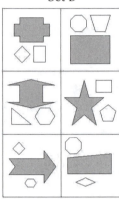

Test shapes

| Question 31 | Question 32 | Question 33 | Question 34 | Question 35 |

Questions 36 to 40

Set A

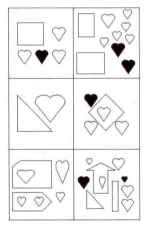

Set B

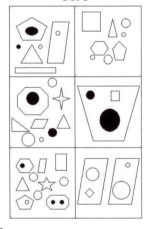

Test shapes

| Question 36 | Question 37 | Question 38 | Question 39 | Question 40 |

Questions 41 to 45

Set A

Set B

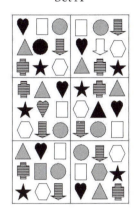
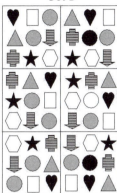

Test shapes

Question 41	Question 42	Question 43	Question 44	Question 45

Questions 46 to 50

Set A

Set B

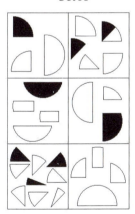
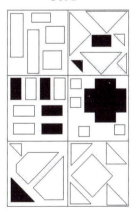

Test shapes

Question 46	Question 47	Question 48	Question 49	Question 50

Questions 51 to 55

Set A

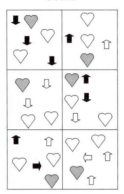

Set B

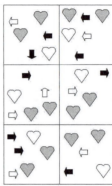

Test shapes

| Question 51 | Question 52 | Question 53 | Question 54 | Question 55 |

Questions 56 to 60

Set A

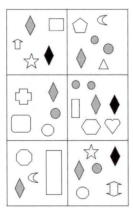

Set B

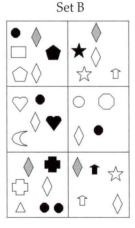

Test shapes

| Question 56 | Question 57 | Question 58 | Question 59 | Question 60 |

Questions 61 to 65

Set A

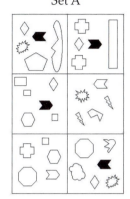

Set B

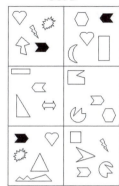

Test shapes

Question 61	Question 62	Question 63	Question 64	Question 65

 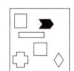 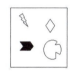

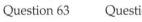
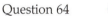

Chapter 8
Decision Analysis practice subtest 2

The Decision Analysis subtest is an on-screen test that consists of one scenario and 26 associated items. The scenario may contain text, tables and other types of information. The 26 items have four or five response options and for some items more than one of the options may be correct. Where more than one of the response options is correct this is clearly identified within the item. A period of thirty minutes is allowed for the test, with one minute for instruction and the remaining twenty-nine minutes for items.

The answers and rationale for this subtest can be found on page 179.

The Mesopotamian codes

In the early part of the 19th century a cache of codes was discovered that had been used across the Mesopotamian empire towards the end of the 6th century when other countries were emerging in the Middle East. These codes substantially consisted of letters and numbers of Greek and Cyrillic origin. Together with the cache of codes there was also a number of actual coded messages and from these the code's structure was determined. The codes were used for political and military purposes and also social insurrection. The information from the codes may not always be complete, but you are asked to make your 'best judgement' based on this information and not on what you might consider to be reasonable.

Table: The Mesopotamian codes

Political codes	Military codes	Social codes	Other codes
Σ = government	123 = Mongolia	Я = peace	β = unlawful
T = police	213 = Greece	Г = terrorists	γ = comparison
U = budget	231 = Mesopotamia	Ђ = conscription	δ = converse
φ = opposition	312 = Persia	Љ = rich	¥ = combine
λ = transport	Э = allies	999 = weak	ə = opposite
ψ = meeting	κ = gunpowder	666 = public	η = less
χ = health	λλ = secret	333 = inside	œ = greater
010 = policy	Ю = war	Z = people	+ = negative
101 = housing	Ж = insurgents	E = include	= = achieve
110 = employment	Ф = attack	π = female	~ = day
	Ω = army		

Question 1

What is the best interpretation of the following coded message:
312, 213 Z, œ, U, 123, Ω

A. The Greek army budget is greater than that of Persia or Mongolia.

B. Persia and Mongolia have smaller armies than Greece.

C. The Greek army budget is greater than that of Persia but is smaller than that of Mongolia.

D. Greece is greater than Persia or Mongolia due to its army.

E. The Greek army budget is less than that of Persia or Mongolia.

Question 2

What is the best interpretation of the following coded message:
Ω, + 110, ǝ π, 231, Ђ

A. Conscription is compulsory for men in Mesopotamia.

B. Unemployed men are forced to join the Mesopotamia army.

C. Women are employed in the Mesopotamian army.

D. Mesopotamia uses conscription to battle unemployment.

E. Unemployed women do not have to join the Mesopotamian army.

Question 3

What is the best interpretation of the following coded message:
Σ,(¥ Φ œ), 101 η, Ж, Γ' Z

A. Insurgents attacked the terrorist group at government house.

B. Government insurgents attacked the terrorist group.

C. Government house was invaded by terrorists and insurgents.

D. Terrorist groups took over government house during the attack.

E. Terrorist groups and insurgents attacked government house.

Question 4

What is the best interpretation of the following coded message:
η, Ω, Γ', β, T, 999 œ

A. The army and the police were no match for the terrorists.

B. Unlawful attacks were made on the police and the army.

C. Terrorists broke the law and the police were powerless without the army.

D. Terrorists have illegally joined the army and the police.

E. Unlawful terrorists attacked the army and the police.

Question 5

What is the best interpretation of the following coded message:
231, Z, χ +, œ + Љ

A. The population of Mesopotamia are healthy and rich.

B. Mesopotamia is a poor and unhealthy country.

C. The population of Mesopotamia suffer from absolute poverty.

D. Suffering and poverty are widespread in Mesopotamia.

E. The people of Mesopotamia are healthy but very poor.

Question 6

What is the best interpretation of the following coded message:
U, η, Σ, κ, 010 œ, 101, 110, (123 312 213 231)

A. The governments of all countries are cutting housing budgets during this volatile time.

B. The governments of Persia, Mongolia and Greece are cutting housing budgets.

C. Jobs will be lost in all countries and building will cease due to a loss of budget.

D. Politically explosive policies on housing and jobs will cut budgets in all countries.

E. Governments of all countries will face political and economic challenges.

Question 7

What is the best interpretation of the following coded message:
Ω, Ω, 333, Ж œ, δ, λλ, ψ

A. The army are having a meeting behind closed doors to discuss insurgency within the ranks.

B. Insurgents have secretly attended army meetings and this has conversely affected security.

C. Insurgents are to be found within in all ranks of the armed forces therefore meetings are held in secret.

D. The army is going to hold a secret meeting with the insurgents to discuss a way forward.

E. High ranking members of the army are holding a secret meeting with the insurgents.

Question 8

What is the best interpretation of the following coded message:
¥ (Я Z), ψ, ¥(ə 666), λλ, T

A. The secret police prevent people demonstrating for peace.

B. The public protest against the war and the secret police.

C. The secret police permit people to hold public meetings.

D. People want peace and hold secret meetings with the police.

E. Pacifists meet in private to avoid the secret police.

Question 9

Which **two** of the following would be the most useful additions to the codes when attempting to convey the following message:

Mesopotamia signed a peace treaty with Persia agreeing to release all enemy prisoners.

A. confine

B. capture

C. concur

D. write

E detainees

Question 10

What is the best interpretation of the following coded message:
Σ, η, U , Z, χ, γ, Ω

A. The government spending on health compares with that of the army.

B. The money raised from the people provides a strong army.

C. The government spending on the army exceeds that spent on citizens' health.

D. The health of the population is important to the government.

E. The government has both a health and military budget.

Question 11

What is the best interpretation of the following coded message:
Ω, Σ, 010, 123, ¥(œ Φ), ¥(γ Γ)

A. The Mongolian government's policy is to execute all terrorists.

B. The Mongolian government and army undertake concerted attacks on terrorists.

C. A military junta is in charge in Mongolia and deals brutally with acts of disaffection.

D. The army and government of Mongolia deal savagely with insurgents.

E. The Mongolian military junta trains its own terrorists in the art of war.

Question 12

What would be the best way to encode the following message:

Persia won the war with Mongolia and they are now our strong allies.

A. 312, œ, Ю, 123, Э, ¥(η Ω)

B. 312, =, Ю, 123, ¥(γ ~), ¥(ә , 999), Э

C. 312, =, δ, ψ, 123, ~, ¥(γ η), Ω

D. 312, œ, ә , 123, ¥(ә 999), Э

E. 312, =, Ю, 123, ¥(γ ~), ¥(γ η), Э

Question 13

What is the best interpretation of the following coded message:
213, ¥(γ δ), Ю, 231

A. The Mesopotamian army attacks the Greek army.

B. The Greek army is under attack from the Mesopotamian army.

C. Mesopotamia at war with Greece.

D. Greece declares war on Mesopotamia.

E. Mesopotamia is under attack from the Greek army.

Question 14

What is the best interpretation of the following coded message:
213, 010, ¥(η β), β, 101, κ, ¥(ə E), Ω, Z

A. Greece requires all stores of gunpowder to be surrendered by both the military and the population.

B. It is unlawful in Greece for any person, military or civilian, to store gunpowder.

C. Greece is clamping down on armed terrorists' use of explosives.

D. It is against Greek law to be in possession of gunpowder without authority.

E. Greece passed a law forbidding the storage of explosives except by military personnel.

Question 15

What is the best interpretation of the following coded message:
213, δ, ¥(ə ~), ¥(β Z ψ), 333, 213

A. Greece declares a night-time curfew across the country.

B. Greeks have declared that a curfew imposed by the government is unlawful.

C. Greece subjects all non-Greeks to a night-time curfew.

D. Greeks who have a criminal conviction are subject to a night-time curfew.

E. Greece's night-time curfew excludes the native Greek population.

Question 16

What is the best interpretation of the following coded message:
123, 213, 110, Γ, ¥(ə 333 123 213), œ, ¥(123 213 Ω)

A. Terrorists from Middle Eastern countries often infiltrate the enemy's armed forces.

B. Mongolia and Greece make use of terrorists from other countries to increase the size of their armies.

C. Terrorists from Mongolia and Greece are trained to fight by their respective armies.

D. Mongolia and Greece have a pact that terrorists from their countries will not attack each other's army.

E. Terrorists of Mongolian and Greek origin mainly commit acts of terrorism against the armed forces of their own country.

Question 17

What would be the best way to encode the following message:

Persia is demanding that some Greek soldiers face war crime charges.

A.   312, ¥(ə δ), 213, Ω, Z, Ж, ¥(Ф Ю β)

B.   312, ¥(ə δ), 213, Ω, Z, Г, Ф, Ю, β

C.   312, ¥(ə, 999, δ), 213, Ω, Z, ¥(Ю β Ф)

D.   312, ¥(ə δ), 213, Ω, Z, Г, β, Ф

E.   312, ¥(ə 999), δ, 213, Ω, Ж, ¥(Ю β Ф)

Question 18

What is the best interpretation of the following coded message:
Z, 312, Я, ψ, ¥(ə η), Ф, γ(Ф T)

A.   The Persian people are a peace-loving nation though they are subjected to marshal law.

B.   People in Persia are not used to peace, having problems with insurgents and a brutal police force.

C.   The Persian people are often harassed by the police without just cause.

D.   People in Persia holding peaceful demonstrations are often fired on by riot police.

E.   The Persian people are law abiding and know the police will crack down on any dissent.

Question 19

What is the best interpretation of the following coded message:
¥(η ~), Ж, κ, 213, Σ, 101, ¥(œ Z), ¥(œ Ф)

A.   Today in the Greek parliament there was an explosion believed to be caused by terrorists killing several people.

B.   Members of the Greek government exploded over the recent killing of some of its ministers.

C.   Insurgents are believed responsible for a bomb that killed a minister and several others in the Greek parliament building.

D.   Recently a bomb was planted in the Greek parliament building that could have killed hundreds of people.

E.   Yesterday insurgents blew up the Greek parliament building and a large number of people were killed.

Question 20

What is the best interpretation of the following coded message:
¥(+ 123 213 231 312), Φ, ¥(123 213 231 312), +, =

A. People from outside Mongolia, Greece, Mesopotamia and Persia often fight as mercenaries for these countries.

B. Mongolia, Greece, Mesopotamia and Persia are often at war with each other.

C. Other countries sometimes fight alongside Mongolia, Greece, Mesopotamia or Persia to help them win.

D. Mongolia, Greece, Mesopotamia and Persia have often defeated other countries.

E. Other countries sometimes invade the Middle East but without success.

Question 21

What is the best interpretation of the following coded message:
γ(E Ю), ¥(œ Z Φ), 213, Ю, 231, π, δ(œ Z)

A. In the war between Greece and Mesopotamia the most significant casualties were civilians.

B. Like all wars women and children were used to fight in the war between Greece and Mesopotamia.

C. Comparatively the number of people killed in the war between Greece and Mesopotamia were mainly civilians.

D. As with all wars the main casualties when Greece fought Mesopotamia were women and children.

E. In comparison to other wars there were a large number of females killed in the war between Greece and Mesopotamia.

Question 22

What is the best interpretation of the following coded message:
123, λλ, T, γ(Φ Z), ¥(+ Σ), ¥(+ =), Ω, Σ, ¥(γ Φ)

A. The Mongolian secret police are rounding up dissidents to prevent the military government being overthrown.

B. Mongolian police are devising secret plans to detain people known to oppose the government.

C. The military police of Mongolia are helping in the overthrow of insurgents infiltrating the government.

D. The Mongolian secret police have discovered a large-scale plan to destabilise the current government.

E. Mongolian police have discovered an underground network of people determined to overthrow the government.

Question 23

Which **two** of the following would be the most useful additions to the codes when attempting to convey the following message:

To safeguard its borders Greece often came to Mesopotamia's assistance during its wars with Mongolia.

A. help

B. boundary

C. frequent

D. protect

E. restore

Question 24

What is the best interpretation of the following coded message:
¥(Z 312 Σ), Э, γ(Γ Z), ¥(123 213 231)

A. The people of Persia support their government in clamping down on terrorists from Mongolia, Greece and Mesopotamia.

B. Members of the Persian government have close ties with different terrorist groups in other countries.

C. The Persian population has its own terrorists just like those in Mongolia, Greece and Mesopotamia.

D. The people that govern Persia are looking at different ways of dealing with terrorists from other countries.

E. Persia is trying to ally itself with the terrorist groups operating in Mongolia, Greece and Mesopotamia.

Question 25

What are the **two** best interpretations of the following coded message:
231, Ω, œ, 123, Ω, γ, 312, Ω, +, œ, 213, Ω

A. The Mesopotamian army is bigger than the Mongolian army, comparative to the Persian army, but not as big as the Greek army.

B. The Mongolian army is bigger than the Persian army.

C. The Persian army is smaller than both the Mongolian and the Mesopotamian armies.

D. The Mongolian army is the second smallest army in the Middle East.

E. Greece's army is bigger than those of Mesopotamia, Mongolia or Persia.

Question 26

What is the best interpretation of the following coded message:
¥(γ Я), ¥(+ Ю), δ, œ, 213

A. War and peace have been a part of Greece's legacy.

B. Peace has been declared after a long war with Greece.

C. Make love not war was a phrase used by the ancient Greeks.

D. The Greeks have had enough of war and are suing for peace.

E. The majority of Greeks want peace not war.

Part III
Non-Cognitive Analysis
practice test

Chapter 9
Non-Cognitive Analysis practice subtest

In 2011 the UKCAT Consortium decided that candidates would not be required to take the Non-Cognitive Analysis subtest (the behavioural test). However, the Consortium have stated on their website that this test '…will be reintroduced into future years of testing after further research has taken place on the use of these scores.' As a result of this action consideration was given to the removal of the chapter but it was decided to retain it because the date of reintroduction of the behavioural test is not known.

The Non-Cognitive Analysis subtest is an on-screen test that consists of a series of questions where aspects of your empathy, integrity and honesty or robustness are being assessed. A period of thirty minutes is allowed for the test. The actual number of questions is not given by the examining body but normally this type of test would contain somewhere between 100 and 160 questions in the timescale allowed. The following test contains 160 questions.

The subtest contains three distinctive styles of questions.

The first style relates to questions that cover a range of behaviours, attitudes, experiences, reactions to stress and feelings of well-being. You will be asked to indicate how strongly you agree with each statement. There are no right or wrong answers. However, note that in the actual examination there may be a variation on indicating how strongly you agree with a statement where you will be asked how well a statement describes you or how true it is of you.

The second style relates to questions that describe situations where you have to decide what to do according to your opinions and values. Again there are no right or wrong answers. Rather, you are asked to choose an answer from a series of options that most closely reflects your value system and what you believe is appropriate in each situation.

The third style consists of paired statements that represent opposing points of view. Read each set and identify your agreement within the six-point range between the statements.

Essentially, the Non-Cognitive Analysis subtest is a personality test and as such there are no correct answers. However, 'preferred answers' have been provided in Part IV of the book, though it must be stressed that these are the preferred answers of the authors and you may well find your responses are different. 'Integrity' and 'honesty' have been taken as synonymous terms and all relevant answers refer to 'integrity' only.

The answers and rationale for this subtest can be found on page 187.

The following statements cover a range of behaviour, attitudes, experiences, reactions to stress and feelings of well-being. You are asked to indicate how strongly you agree or disagree with each statement. For example, if you strongly agree with first statement 'I can get annoyed when I have to work late' you would circle option 'A' Strongly Agree. There are no right or wrong answers.

1. I can get annoyed when I have to work late.

   A. Strongly Agree   B. Agree   C. Disagree   (D) Strongly Disagree

2. If you look and sound intelligent others will respect you.

   A. Strongly Agree   B. Agree   (C) Disagree   D. Strongly Disagree

3. I avoid losing my temper with others.

   A. Strongly Agree   (B) Agree   C. Disagree   D. Strongly Disagree

4. I think it is important to exercise regularly.

   (A) Strongly Agree   B. Agree   C. Disagree   D. Strongly Disagree

5. It is important to move in the right social circles to get yourself noticed.

   A. Strongly Agree   B. Agree   C. Disagree   (D) Strongly Disagree

6. I understand why people sometimes do bad things.

   A. Strongly Agree   (B) Agree   C. Disagree   D. Strongly Disagree

7. Stress is just a part of everyday working life.

   A. Strongly Agree   (B) Agree   C. Disagree   D. Strongly Disagree

8. We all make mistakes and should own up to them.

   (A) Strongly Agree   B. Agree   C. Disagree   D. Strongly Disagree

9. I would not resort to violence even when aggravated.

   (A) Strongly Agree   B. Agree   C. Disagree   D. Strongly Disagree

10. I am always happy to meet challenges head-on.

    (A) Strongly Agree   B. Agree   C. Disagree   D. Strongly Disagree

11. People always have a right to be told the truth even if it hurts.

    (A) Strongly Agree   B. Agree   C. Disagree   D. Strongly Disagree

♭ 12. I am tolerant when anxious people feel the need to talk.

    (A.) Strongly Agree   B. Agree   C. Disagree   D. Strongly Disagree

C 13. I seldom lose an argument.

    A. Strongly Agree   (B.) Agree   C. Disagree   D. Strongly Disagree

14. Loyalty to your employer is sacrosanct.

    A. Strongly Agree   B. Agree   (C.) Disagree   D. Strongly Disagree

15. I can cope when distressed people are abusive.

    A. Strongly Agree   (B.) Agree   C. Disagree   D. Strongly Disagree

16. People can sometimes expect too much from you.

    A. Strongly Agree   (B.) Agree   C. Disagree   D. Strongly Disagree

β 17. I'm not perfect and tell people if I don't know something.

    (A.) Strongly Agree   B. Agree   C. Disagree   D. Strongly Disagree

β 18. Sometimes it is necessary to show a gentle side.

    (A.) Strongly Agree   B. Agree   C. Disagree   D. Strongly Disagree

19. I believe being strong-minded is an asset.

    A. Strongly Agree   (B.) Agree   C. Disagree   D. Strongly Disagree

20. I have occasionally pretended to be something that I'm not.

    A. Strongly Agree   B. Agree   C. Disagree   (D.) Strongly Disagree

21. If someone hurts me I sometimes feel the need to retaliate.

    A. Strongly Agree   B. Agree   (C.) Disagree   D. Strongly Disagree

C 22. I sometimes feel tense when I have too much work.

    A. Strongly Agree   (B.) Agree   C. Disagree   D. Strongly Disagree

23. I believe sincerity to be a virtue.

    (A.) Strongly Agree   B. Agree   C. Disagree   D. Strongly Disagree

24. I can be sensitive and intuitive when dealing with others.

    (A.) Strongly Agree   B. Agree   C. Disagree   D. Strongly Disagree

25. It is important to vigorously defend peoples' rights.

    A. Strongly Agree   (B.) Agree   C. Disagree   D. Strongly Disagree

26. Some people don't deserve the help they receive.

    A. Strongly Agree   B. Agree   (C.) Disagree   D. Strongly Disagree

27. Humanitarian issues stir me.

    (A.) Strongly Agree   B. Agree   C. Disagree   D. Strongly Disagree

28. I find that giving people bad news is really hard.

    A. Strongly Agree   (B.) Agree   C. Disagree   D. Strongly Disagree

29. I am always genuinely concerned about others' feelings.

    (A.) Strongly Agree   B. Agree   C. Disagree   D. Strongly Disagree

30. I handle traumatic information in a sensitive manner.

    A. Strongly Agree   (B.) Agree   C. Disagree   D. Strongly Disagree

31. Inflicting pain on others can be a necessary evil.

    A. Strongly Agree   (B.) Agree   C. Disagree   D. Strongly Disagree

32. You can't always be honest with people especially when it's going to hurt their feelings.

    A. Strongly Agree   B. Agree   C. Disagree   (D.) Strongly Disagree

33. I respect and value the views of others.

    (A.) Strongly Agree   B. Agree   C. Disagree   D. Strongly Disagree

34. A healthy body means a healthy mind.

    (A.) Strongly Agree   B. Agree   C. Disagree   D. Strongly Disagree

35. I like to be frank with people and not beat about the bush.

    A. Strongly Agree   (B.) Agree   C. Disagree   D. Strongly Disagree

36. I sometimes get impatient when discussing issues with people who have difficulty understanding.

    A. Strongly Agree   B. Agree   C. Disagree   D. Strongly Disagree

37. Some people don't know best and have to accept what I say.

    A. Strongly Agree   B. Agree   C. Disagree   D. Strongly Disagree

38. I am a better person than someone with low integrity.

A. Strongly Agree   B. Agree   C. Disagree   D. Strongly Disagree

39. It is important to accept individual lifestyle differences.

A. Strongly Agree   B. Agree   C. Disagree   D. Strongly Disagree

40. People need to deal with work stress and get on with it.

A. Strongly Agree   B. Agree   C. Disagree   D. Strongly Disagree

41. People who take things from work should be prosecuted or sacked.

A. Strongly Agree   B. Agree   C. Disagree   D. Strongly Disagree

42. I take account of the feelings of others.

A. Strongly Agree   B. Agree   C. Disagree   D. Strongly Disagree

43. I have taken umbrage at having to work long hours.

A. Strongly Agree   B. Agree   C. Disagree   D. Strongly Disagree

44. I'm different at work from how I am socially.

A. Strongly Agree   B. Agree   C. Disagree   D. Strongly Disagree

45. I understand when people are distressed.

A. Strongly Agree   B. Agree   C. Disagree   D. Strongly Disagree

46. I have occasionally done more exercise than was good for me.

A. Strongly Agree   B. Agree   C. Disagree   D. Strongly Disagree

47. You should never pretend there is always a happy ending.

A. Strongly Agree   B. Agree   C. Disagree   D. Strongly Disagree

48. I believe it is possible to remain patient with difficult people.

A. Strongly Agree   B. Agree   C. Disagree   D. Strongly Disagree

49. I can get upset when something I've done well is ignored.

A. Strongly Agree   B. Agree   C. Disagree   D. Strongly Disagree

50. If I find anything I always hand it in to the appropriate authority.

A. Strongly Agree   B. Agree   C. Disagree   D. Strongly Disagree

51. I understand when people feel they have suffered too much.

    A. Strongly Agree   B. Agree   C. Disagree   D. Strongly Disagree

52. I find I can detach myself from other people's grief.

    A. Strongly Agree   B. Agree   C. Disagree   D. Strongly Disagree

53. I can understand why world events make people xenophobic.

    A. Strongly Agree   B. Agree   C. Disagree   D. Strongly Disagree

54. I take account of views that are radically different from mine.

    A. Strongly Agree   B. Agree   C. Disagree   D. Strongly Disagree

55. It is important to show you're confident even when you feel inadequate.

    A. Strongly Agree   B. Agree   C. Disagree   D. Strongly Disagree

56. People in positions of authority who accept bribes should always be prosecuted.

    A. Strongly Agree   B. Agree   C. Disagree   D. Strongly Disagree

57. Everyone, no matter what their problems, has a right to be treated the same.

    A. Strongly Agree   B. Agree   C. Disagree   D. Strongly Disagree

58. How you say something is sometimes more important than what you say.

    A. Strongly Agree   B. Agree   C. Disagree   D. Strongly Disagree

59. I often have difficulty with people in authority.

    A. Strongly Agree   B. Agree   C. Disagree   D. Strongly Disagree

60. The problems caused by addictions should be sensitively handled.

    A. Strongly Agree   B. Agree   C. Disagree   D. Strongly Disagree

61. There are hardships in every walk of life and you just have to get on with it.

    A. Strongly Agree   B. Agree   C. Disagree   D. Strongly Disagree

62. I rarely say anything that I don't really mean.

    A. Strongly Agree   B. Agree   C. Disagree   D. Strongly Disagree

63. Birth control and abortion are and should be a personal decision.

    A. Strongly Agree   B. Agree   C. Disagree   D. Strongly Disagree

64. I have always been uneasy in large social gatherings.

    A. Strongly Agree   B. Agree   C. Disagree   D. Strongly Disagree

65. You should always find someone to blame when a mistake has been made.

    A. Strongly Agree   B. Agree   C. Disagree   D. Strongly Disagree

66. Casualties from any side of any war should be treated equally.

    A. Strongly Agree   B. Agree   C. Disagree   D. Strongly Disagree

67. If I don't know how to do something I ask someone else who does.

    A. Strongly Agree   B. Agree   C. Disagree   D. Strongly Disagree

68. I think swearing in the workplace is just indicative of where society is at.

    A. Strongly Agree   B. Agree   C. Disagree   D. Strongly Disagree

69. I fully support the work of those dealing with mental illness.

    A. Strongly Agree   B. Agree   C. Disagree   D. Strongly Disagree

70. I have learnt to cope with the strain of having too much on my plate.

    A. Strongly Agree   B. Agree   C. Disagree   D. Strongly Disagree

71. Dishonesty is acceptable in certain circumstances.

    A. Strongly Agree   B. Agree   C. Disagree   D. Strongly Disagree

72. Too much emphasis is placed on the rehabilitation of offenders.

    A. Strongly Agree   B. Agree   C. Disagree   D. Strongly Disagree

73. I sometimes resent people who are more popular than I am.

    A. Strongly Agree   B. Agree   C. Disagree   D. Strongly Disagree

74. Being a professional person I should be a role model for others.

    A. Strongly Agree   B. Agree   C. Disagree   D. Strongly Disagree

75. It is important to respect the beliefs of others.

    A. Strongly Agree   B. Agree   C. Disagree   D. Strongly Disagree

76. I find it easy to cope with people's high expectations of my work.

    A. Strongly Agree   B. Agree   C. Disagree   D. Strongly Disagree

77. There are occasions where it is best not to be too honest with people.

    A. Strongly Agree   B. Agree   C. Disagree   D. Strongly Disagree

78. It is better to be a good listener than talker.

    A. Strongly Agree   B. Agree   C. Disagree   D. Strongly Disagree

79. I like the person I have become.

    A. Strongly Agree   B. Agree   C. Disagree   D. Strongly Disagree

80. I would happily defend anyone who had a genuine grievance.

    A. Strongly Agree   B. Agree   C. Disagree   D. Strongly Disagree

81. An injured drunk driver should be treated sensitively.

    A. Strongly Agree   B. Agree   C. Disagree   D. Strongly Disagree

82. When I have made a mistake I just want to run and hide.

    A. Strongly Agree   B. Agree   C. Disagree   D. Strongly Disagree

83. I believe that secrets are sometimes compatible with professional behaviour.

    A. Strongly Agree   B. Agree   C. Disagree   D. Strongly Disagree

84. People who give their time to charities are commendable.

    A. Strongly Agree   B. Agree   C. Disagree   D. Strongly Disagree

85. If you can do it you don't shout it from the rooftops.

    A. Strongly Agree   B. Agree   C. Disagree   D. Strongly Disagree

86. I can understand why some people are deceitful or dishonest.

    A. Strongly Agree   B. Agree   C. Disagree   D. Strongly Disagree

87. It is important to recognise that people have a breaking point.

    A. Strongly Agree   B. Agree   C. Disagree   D. Strongly Disagree

88. I always set myself clear goals and more often than not achieve them.

    A. Strongly Agree   B. Agree   C. Disagree   D. Strongly Disagree

89. I don't suffer fools gladly.

    A. Strongly Agree   B. Agree   C. Disagree   D. Strongly Disagree

90. The lack of good funded care for the elderly is distressing.

    A. Strongly Agree   B. Agree   C. Disagree   D. Strongly Disagree

91. I often get agitated by people who think they know everything.

    A. Strongly Agree   B. Agree   C. Disagree   D. Strongly Disagree

92. Probity in any profession is imperative.

    A. Strongly Agree   B. Agree   C. Disagree   D. Strongly Disagree

93. Hostility and anger can be indicative of emotional trauma.

    A. Strongly Agree   B. Agree   C. Disagree   D. Strongly Disagree

94. I do not like upsetting other people and wherever possible I avoid it.

    A. Strongly Agree   B. Agree   C. Disagree   D. Strongly Disagree

95. It is important to work within the rules of your organisation.

    A. Strongly Agree   B. Agree   C. Disagree   D. Strongly Disagree

96. I feel for those who have to wait for vital treatment.

    A. Strongly Agree   B. Agree   C. Disagree   D. Strongly Disagree

97. I find it easy to talk to other people and make friends.

    A. Strongly Agree   B. Agree   C. Disagree   D. Strongly Disagree

98. I have blamed other people for my mistakes.

    A. Strongly Agree   B. Agree   C. Disagree   D. Strongly Disagree

99. Dying with dignity is important.

    A. Strongly Agree   B. Agree   C. Disagree   D. Strongly Disagree

100. People who want to be the centre of attention often annoy me.

    A. Strongly Agree   B. Agree   C. Disagree   D. Strongly Disagree

101. I think you should be true to yourself and not what others want you to be.

    A. Strongly Agree   B. Agree   C. Disagree   D. Strongly Disagree

102. I can understand why visiting rules in hospitals can cause distress.

    A. Strongly Agree   B. Agree   C. Disagree   D. Strongly Disagree

103. Keeping your own counsel can be beneficial in the long term.

    A. Strongly Agree   B. Agree   C. Disagree   D. Strongly Disagree

104. I believe in the philosophy of 'live and let live'.

    A. Strongly Agree   B. Agree   C. Disagree   D. Strongly Disagree

105. The feelings of the bereaved are foremost when pronouncing death.

    A. Strongly Agree   B. Agree   C. Disagree   D. Strongly Disagree

106. I often become anxious about other people's expectations of my abilities.

    A. Strongly Agree   B. Agree   C. Disagree   D. Strongly Disagree

107. People can tell if you're not being genuine.

    A. Strongly Agree   B. Agree   C. Disagree   D. Strongly Disagree

108. I would be frustrated if I had to wait longer for an operation than others.

    A. Strongly Agree   B. Agree   C. Disagree   D. Strongly Disagree

109. I believe I am as good as, if not better than, most people.

    A. Strongly Agree   B. Agree   C. Disagree   D. Strongly Disagree

110. I believe professional people have a duty to conduct themselves properly both at work and socially.

    A. Strongly Agree   B. Agree   C. Disagree   D. Strongly Disagree

111. Anxious family and friends should be treated sensitively.

    A. Strongly Agree   B. Agree   C. Disagree   D. Strongly Disagree

112. I'd rather people find out for themselves what I'm capable of.

    A. Strongly Agree   B. Agree   C. Disagree   D. Strongly Disagree

113. I think you should always strive to be an upright citizen.

    A. Strongly Agree   B. Agree   C. Disagree   D. Strongly Disagree

114. We may all experience the pressure of work.

    A. Strongly Agree   B. Agree   C. Disagree   D. Strongly Disagree

115. I sometimes get angry when people don't know what they are talking about.

    A. Strongly Agree   B. Agree   C. Disagree   D. Strongly Disagree

116. Being a professional, I am in a better position to know what's right and wrong.

A. Strongly Agree   B. Agree   C. Disagree   D. Strongly Disagree

117. People who have abused their health have as much right to receive treatment.

A. Strongly Agree   B. Agree   C. Disagree   D. Strongly Disagree

118. I make it quite clear if I don't agree with someone's point of view.

A. Strongly Agree   B. Agree   C. Disagree   D. Strongly Disagree

119. I would rather say nothing if I couldn't be straightforward with someone.

A. Strongly Agree   B. Agree   C. Disagree   D. Strongly Disagree

120. I may disagree with others but I am willing to accept their points of view.

A. Strongly Agree   B. Agree   C. Disagree   D. Strongly Disagree

121. I don't find it that easy to confront people when they've done something wrong.

A. Strongly Agree   B. Agree   C. Disagree   D. Strongly Disagree

122. People want you to be open and honest with them.

A. Strongly Agree   B. Agree   C. Disagree   D. Strongly Disagree

123. A calm and friendly manner is positive in difficult situations.

A. Strongly Agree   B. Agree   C. Disagree   D. Strongly Disagree

124. I'm very much a loner and prefer my own company.

A. Strongly Agree   B. Agree   C. Disagree   D. Strongly Disagree

125. You sometimes can't get a job done because of minor health and safety rules.

A. Strongly Agree   B. Agree   C. Disagree   D. Strongly Disagree

126. The elderly need a lot of care, attention and understanding.

A. Strongly Agree   B. Agree   C. Disagree   D. Strongly Disagree

127. People who talk about how good they are at work can often be the opposite.

A. Strongly Agree   B. Agree   C. Disagree   D. Strongly Disagree

128. If I do something I do it to the best of my ability.

A. Strongly Agree   B. Agree   C. Disagree   D. Strongly Disagree

129. Even when death is inevitable it is still difficult for people to come to terms with it.

A. Strongly Agree   B. Agree   C. Disagree   D. Strongly Disagree

130. I find it hard to leave problems at work and often take them home with me.

A. Strongly Agree   B. Agree   C. Disagree   D. Strongly Disagree

131. I frequently check the work I have done.

A. Strongly Agree   B. Agree   C. Disagree   D. Strongly Disagree

132. I understand the anxieties of those awaiting transplant operations.

A. Strongly Agree   B. Agree   C. Disagree   D. Strongly Disagree

133. It is important to stay positive even when it feels like everything that could go wrong has gone wrong.

A. Strongly Agree   B. Agree   C. Disagree   D. Strongly Disagree

134. I have often been accused of being a rebel.

A. Strongly Agree   B. Agree   C. Disagree   D. Strongly Disagree

135. Bereavement counselling is a total waste of time.

A. Strongly Agree   B. Agree   C. Disagree   D. Strongly Disagree

136. It is best not to be top dog as when you're number one there's only one way to go – down.

A. Strongly Agree   B. Agree   C. Disagree   D. Strongly Disagree

137. I always aspire to get things right when I'm at work.

A. Strongly Agree   B. Agree   C. Disagree   D. Strongly Disagree

138. The decision made by parents not to donate their deceased child's organs should be respected.

A. Strongly Agree   B. Agree   C. Disagree   D. Strongly Disagree

139. When I'm feeling really low I don't let on to other people.

A. Strongly Agree   B. Agree   C. Disagree   D. Strongly Disagree

140. I think people in authority often don't understand what's really going on in the workplace.

    A. Strongly Agree   B. Agree   C. Disagree   D. Strongly Disagree

141. One should try to understand when strong beliefs appear counter to our own.

    A. Strongly Agree   B. Agree   C. Disagree   D. Strongly Disagree

142. I often wish I could be somebody else.

    A. Strongly Agree   B. Agree   C. Disagree   D. Strongly Disagree

143. If I have been undercharged in a restaurant I always point this out.

    A. Strongly Agree   B. Agree   C. Disagree   D. Strongly Disagree

144. We can all experience irrational fears or thoughts.

    A. Strongly Agree   B. Agree   C. Disagree   D. Strongly Disagree

145. I have difficulty with people who don't pull their weight.

    A. Strongly Agree   B. Agree   C. Disagree   D. Strongly Disagree

146. Systems and procedures should always be adhered to.

    A. Strongly Agree   B. Agree   C. Disagree   D. Strongly Disagree

147. If people knew me they would say I'd make a good counsellor.

    A. Strongly Agree   B. Agree   C. Disagree   D. Strongly Disagree

148. You should never be too modest about your achievements.

    A. Strongly Agree   B. Agree   C. Disagree   D. Strongly Disagree

149. Expediency can always be used as an excuse to break the rules.

    A. Strongly Agree   B. Agree   C. Disagree   D. Strongly Disagree

150. One needs to be tough and pragmatic, not understanding and sensitive.

    A. Strongly Agree   B. Agree   C. Disagree   D. Strongly Disagree

The following extract describes a situation where you have to decide what to do according to your opinions and values. There are no right or wrong answers. Rather, you are asked to choose an answer from a series of options that most closely reflect your value system and what you believe is appropriate in each situation.

The Company Conundrum

After finishing university you commence work as an engineer with a multi-million pound organisation based in a large office complex in central London.

After a few months you realise that your colleagues, some of whom are friends from university, claim for more hours than they have actually worked. When you confront one of your friends and colleagues about this they tell you that this is normal practice and if you don't show these additional hours, even though you haven't worked them, you could well face dismissal from the company.

Several months later you are spoken to by your supervisor who is concerned at the excessive hours you are working, considering you are relatively new to the company.

What is your opinion? How do you feel about the following statements?

---

151. It is always wrong to deceive an employer.
    A. Strongly Agree   B. Agree   C. Disagree   D. Strongly Disagree

152. It is important to integrate fully with your colleagues even where you may sometimes disagree with their behaviour.
    A. Strongly Agree   B. Agree   C. Disagree   D. Strongly Disagree

153. Friendship always has its boundaries.
    A. Strongly Agree   B. Agree   C. Disagree   D. Strongly Disagree

154. It is important to look at the employer's perspective.
    A. Strongly Agree   B. Agree   C. Disagree   D. Strongly Disagree

155. Honesty is not always the best policy irrespective of the consequences.
    A. Strongly Agree   B. Agree   C. Disagree   D. Strongly Disagree

The following section consists of paired statements that represent opposing points of view. Read each set and identify your agreement within the six-point range between the statements. Scores of 1 to 3 indicate agreement with the first statement and scores of 4 to 6 indicate agreement with the second statement, with 3 or 4 indicating slight agreement with the respective statement, and 1 or 6 indicating strong agreement with the respective statement.

156. I am seldom given a problem that I cannot solve.

1

2

3

4

5

6

I am often given a problem that I have difficulty in solving.

157. I try to adapt my behaviour to the situation.

1

2

3

4

5

6

I think it's important to be who you are in any situation.

158. I always take advice from my friends seriously.

1

2

3

4

5

6

I will always make my own decisions irrespective of others' advice.

159. I have this ability of weighing people up when I first meet them.

1

2

3

4

5

6

It takes time before you really get to know another person.

160. If I'm late for work or an appointment I usually admit I'm in the wrong.

1

2

3

4

5

6

If I'm late for work or an appointment I usually make an excuse.

Part IV
Answers and rationale

Chapter 1
Verbal Reasoning practice subtest 1

Question number	Correct response	Question number	Correct response
1	C	23	A
2	A	24	B
3	B	25	A
4	C	26	C
5	B	27	B
6	A	28	A
7	C	29	A
8	C	30	C
9	C	31	A
10	B	32	B
11	A	33	A
12	C	34	B
13	C	35	C
14	A	36	A
15	B	37	B
16	C	38	C
17	B	39	C
18	B	40	A
19	A	41	A
20	C	42	C
21	C	43	C
22	A	44	A

Passage I: question 1

C. Can't Tell

Although one would assume that being subjected to 'rejection, ridicule or aggression' would affect the recipient's sense of self-worth and overall self-image, this is not actually stated in the passage.

Passage I: question 2

A. True

The 'lack of awareness' is clearly identified in the third sentence of the passage i.e. '...largely based on fear and misunderstanding of what mental health means, and it is not uncommon for questions of capability and risk to be presented as reasons for exclusion. Indirect discrimination is often more complex to identify, as it results from a misunderstanding and adaptation rather than a direct and explicit rejection or exclusion'.

Passage I: question 3

B. False

This is the opposite of what the passage actually states i.e. '... it is not uncommon for questions of capability and risk to be presented as reasons for exclusion.'

Passage I: question 4

C. Can't Tell

Although there is little doubt that in reality this statement is true the passage only makes reference to 'social interaction'. More information would be needed to include 'services, employment and training.'

Passage II: question 5

B. False

The question does not take account of the restrictions relating to 'services where speedy access to diagnosis and treatment are particularly important' (e.g. emergency attendances or admissions).

Passage II: question 6

A. True

It is quite explicit in the passage that 'patients attending a Rapid Access Chest Pain Clinic under the two-week maximum waiting time, and patients attending cancer services under the two-week maximum waiting time' do not qualify for the Choice agenda.

Passage II: question 7

C. Can't Tell

Although the passage specifically relates to GPs in England there may or may not be similar systems in Wales and/or Scotland. Further information would be required to determine this.

Passage II: question 8

C. Can't Tell

Although it might be assumed that Rapid Access Chest Pain Clinics and cancer services are provided by independent and private hospitals, this is not clear in the passage. The passage only states that patients using these services do not qualify for the Choice agenda.

Passage III: question 9

C. Can't Tell

Although the passage states that type 2 diabetes is often associated with obesity and type 2 diabetes is linked with sleeping disorders, further information would be required as the research is only 'suggesting' such a connection.

Passage III: question 10

B. False

The final sentence of the passage states 'The findings of the research will raise the possibility of genetic tests to identify people vulnerable to developing type 2 diabetes'. Therefore these tests are not yet available, and in any case would identify only a potential vulnerability to diabetes, rather than the disease itself.

Passage III: question 11

A. True

The passage states type 2 diabetes affects 'about 2.3 million people in the UK, with at least 500,000 more who are not aware that they have the condition', and adding these together makes 2.8 million people.

Passage III: question 12

C. Can't Tell

Although the passage refers to how the body responds to the '24-hour cycle of light and dark' and 'a hormone that is part of the body's internal clock', there is no actual information about people being awake during the night and sleeping during the day, and further information would be required to authenticate this or otherwise.

Passage IV: question 13

C. Can't Tell

This is a very general statement. Although there may be a profit reduction in relation to some drugs purchased by the Health Service, the paragraph does state 'they will still be able to charge what they want' and therefore without additional information a 'true' or 'false' answer cannot be determined.

Passage IV: question 14

A. True

It is made quite clear in the passage that 'Currently, a number of effective drugs are not used because they are too expensive'. It can be inferred from the rest of the passage that this includes more effective treatments for heart disease and cancer.

Passage IV: question 15

B. False

Drug companies, as with all other private companies, operate in a world where profit ensures their existence and satisfies shareholders. The passage itself states that drug companies will enter negotiations for a 'realistic' value to be agreed but also goes on to say 'they will still be able to charge what they want'.

Passage IV: question 16

C. Can't Tell

Although it might be assumed that there would be a reduction in the death rate from heart disease and cancer, there is no indication of how 'significant' this may be and how this might be measured. Without further information this question cannot be answered in the affirmative or negative.

Passage V: question 17

B. False

It is quite clear that under the new proposals history, geography and science will be 'taught through cross-curriculum themed classes'.

Passage V: question 18

B. False

Although the passage refers to teachers encouraging children's social and emotional well-being to cure some of the 'social ills' facing society, there is nothing in or that can be inferred from the passage about their responsibility for the social fabric of society.

Passage V: question 19

A. True

This is actually stated within the passage: 'It is considered that the teaching of rigid subject areas in primary schools was making children's knowledge and understanding shallow.'

Passage V: question 20

C. Can't Tell

Although this is undoubtedly the desired outcome from the recommended changes, further information will be required over time to assess and compare the children's performance in these subject areas.

Passage VI: question 21

C. Can't Tell

The passage essentially deals with younger children and, although it is suggested that a lack of communication skills will reduce children's chances of educational success, it does not comment on the attainment of educational standards. Further information would be required in relation to this area.

Passage VI: question 22

A. True

This is true as it actually states in the passage that 'in poorer homes children only hear 500 different words a day compared to 1,500 in a better-off household'.

Passage VI: question 23

A. True

This statement can be extrapolated from the passage where it states the following to support the general premise: 'It is believed parents in deprived areas often feel alienated from a child they did not want, may be depressed by their circumstances or not be functioning socially and emotionally because of drugs or alcohol'.

Passage VI: question 24

B. False

The passage states that 'in poorer homes children only hear 500 different words a day compared to 1,500 in a better-off household'. 500 to 1,500 is a ratio of 1:3, therefore children in better-off households are likely to hear three times (not five times) as many different words spoken as those from deprived homes.

Passage VII: question 25

A. True

Although the passage does not directly use the term 'immunisation' this is referred to in the passage as 'artificial immunity (active or passive)'.

Passage VII: question 26

C. Can't Tell

The passage makes no mention of changes in communicable diseases or the emergence of new communicable diseases.

Passage VII: question 27

B. False

The passage states 'The susceptibility of the host is influenced by age, natural immunity, artificial immunity (active or passive), nutritional status and immune suppression' so age, diet and lifestyle choice do have an impact on a person's susceptibility to disease.

Passage VII: question 28

A. True

Although the passage does not specifically state that 'the atmosphere is a vehicle than can carry an infective agent' it does state that 'transmission of infection may be by inhalation' which has the same meaning.

Passage VIII: question 29

A. True

The passage states 'Psychologists and statisticians refer to normal as the middle range of a distribution of values.' The 'middle range' can also be referred to as the 'average' so a lack of significant deviation from the average is 'normal'.

Passage VIII: question 30

C. Can't Tell

The passage states 'A sociologist defines "normal" as that which is in line with a rule for a particular social or cultural group in society.' The statement is suggesting that normality for a particular group may be the violation of norms and standards. The passage does not really provide a definitive answer to this and so more information would be required.

Passage VIII: question 31

A. True

The passage states: 'normal as the most usual' or 'as conforming to a standard' and 'In common speech, "normal" may simply mean "not abnormal, not strange"'. Therefore 'strange' is used as a synonym for 'abnormal,' i.e. not normal.

Passage VIII: question 32

B. False

The passage states 'In medicine "normal" is often used to mean an absence of physiological pathology.' The adverb 'often' is used, which means 'frequently' or 'many times'. The statement uses the word 'everyone' hence the answer is 'false'.

Passage IX: question 33

A. True

This is apparent from the passage, which says that views on the use of Internet technology differ considerably between managers (and especially those under 35) and senior executives.

Passage IX: question 34

B. False

It does not state this in the passage. Internet access was allowed, albeit sometimes restricted. Senior executives were generally pessimistic about some of the benefits, but they still allow Internet access.

Passage IX: question 35

C. Can't Tell

Although it states in the passage that '65% of organisations monitored Internet usage, and this rose to 88% in the police', and it might be assumed that this would be the case because of their accountability, it is not actually stated in the passage and therefore further information would be required to authenticate this as a fact.

Passage IX: question 36

A. True

This item relates to the statement 'Also, 65% blocked access to "inappropriate" sites, with this rising to 89% in local government and 90% in the utilities'. In relation to the '65%' figure it could be said that 35% do not block access to 'inappropriate' Internet sites.

Passage X: question 37

B. False

Workers will be able to work in excess of 48 hours a week as the maximum working hours limit is averaged out over a one-year period.

Passage X: question 38

C. Can't Tell

This may well be the outcome but cannot be stated without further information being provided.

Passage X: question 39

C. Can't Tell

The passage states: 'The trade unions are in favour of the European maximum 48-hour limit'; however, this does not necessarily relate to overtime. It would be possible for overtime to be worked up to the 48-hour limit. Further information would be required to assess the trade unions' position in relation to overtime.

Passage X: question 40

A. True

There is no doubt that this answer is true as in the passage it states: 'The government believe the working hours limit would cost the UK economy tens of billions of pounds over the next 10 years.'

Passage XI: question 41

A. True

The whole tenet of the passage is about the benefit of technology, and not about it being a barrier to learning and especially the benefit in relation to people with disabilities and learning difficulties.

Passage XI: question 42

C. Can't Tell

No information is given in the passage about academic qualifications, so the answer must be Can't Tell.

Passage XI: question 43

C. Can't Tell

Although one might assume that a policy exists in universities for offering students equal learning opportunities, this is not stated in the passage and more information would be required.

Passage XI: question 44

A. True

The ways in which new technology helps students with disabilities and learning difficulties is amply qualified within the passage.

Chapter 2
Quantitative Reasoning practice subtest 1

Question number	Correct response	Question number	Correct response
1	E	19	D
2	B	20	B
3	A	21	D
4	C	22	C
5	D	23	B
6	C	24	A
7	A	25	E
8	E	26	A
9	D	27	A
10	C	28	D
11	D	29	C
12	E	30	E
13	C	31	A
14	D	32	C
15	E	33	B
16	D	34	C
17	B	35	E
18	C	36	A

Question 1

Answer E is correct: 70%

The minimum score required on the on-screen hazard simulation test is 37, and there were 14 respondents who scored 37 or higher. Write this number as a fraction of the total and multiply by 100 to attain the percentage, i.e. $\frac{14}{20} \times 100 = 70\%$.

Question 2

Answer B is correct: 39.

The mode is the number in the distribution that has the highest frequency. In the information relating to females the score of 39 appears twice and every other number only once.

Question 3

Answer A is correct: 21.

The range of a distribution is the difference between the highest and lowest values. The highest value is 44 and the lowest value is 23, therefore 44 – 23 = 21.

Question 4

Answer C is correct: Less than half of the respondents scored above the mean.

To calculate the mean, sum the values of the distribution and divide by the number of values, i.e. $\frac{794}{20}$ = 39.70. The number of scores above the mean is 9, therefore less than half of the respondents scored above the mean.

Question 5

Answer D is correct: 67.5%.

Surface mail would cost: 4 letters at £1.99 = £7.96; 5 × packets less than 500g at £3.65 = £18.25. Total cost £7.96 + £18.25 = £26.21.

Airmail would cost: 4 letters at £9.16 = £36.64; 3 × 200g packets at £8.42 = £25.26; 2 × 300g packets at £9.06 = £18.12 + 56p surcharge = £18.68. Total = £80.58.

Surface mail would be cheaper than airmail as a percentage: Difference between surface and airmail is £80.58 – £26.21 = £54.37, which as a percentage is $\frac{54.37}{80.58}$ × 100 = 67.5%.

Question 6

Answer C is correct: £170.20.

The cost of sending 25 letters each weighing 100g would be 25 × £8.51 = £212.75.

20% of £212.75 is $\frac{212.75}{100}$ × 20 = £42.55.

The cost of sending 25 letters each weighing 100g without VAT would be £212.75 – £42.55 = £170.20.

Question 7

Answer A is correct: Airmail letters weighing 1 kilogram cost an extra £6.60 in addition to the price of a 300g letter.

Airmail letters over 300g, for every 20g up to 500g add 16p, so 200g = 10 × 16p = £1.60; for every 20g up to 1kg add 20p, so 500g = 25 × 20p = £5.00. The extra cost of a 1 kilogram airmail letter is £1.60 + £5.00 = £6.60.

Question 8

Answer E is correct: £158.22

Each letter is of equal weight so calculate the weight of each letter, 4.5 kilograms, or $\frac{4,500}{27} = 166.7g$.

The cost of one 166.7g surface mail letter is £5.86, so the cost of 27 letters is £5.86 × 27 = £158.22.

Question 9

Answer D is correct: 10%.

Calculate the total number of books, write the number of 'history' books as a fraction of the total and multiply by 100 to obtain the percentage, i.e. $\frac{5,700}{55,400}$ × 100 = 10%.

Question 10

Answer C is correct: £5.96

The cost of a fiction paperback is the total stock selling price divided by the number of paperbacks, i.e. $\frac{101,362.50}{12,750}$ = £7.95. The cost of 3 books is £7.95 × 3 = 23.85, therefore $\frac{23.85}{4}$ = £5.96.

Question 11

Answer D is correct: £3,915.50.

The profit is $\frac{1}{3}$ of the selling price. For the total stock it would be $\frac{31,324}{3}$ = £10,441.33. To obtain $\frac{3}{8}$ of the profit , first obtain $\frac{1}{8}$, i.e. $\frac{10,441.33}{8}$ = 1,305.17, and then multiply this by 3, i.e. 1,305.17 × 3 = £3,915.50.

Question 12

Answer E is correct: 10,850.

The range of a distribution is the difference between the highest and lowest values. The highest value is 12,750 and the lowest value is 1,900, therefore the range is 12,750 – 1,900 = 10,850.

Question 13

Answer C is correct: The average number of texts per person for Ireland (Irl) is 2,016 per annum, up from 128 per month five years ago.

To obtain the average number of texts per person for Ireland per annum multiply 168 × 12 = 2,016. To obtain the average number of texts per month 5 years ago: $\frac{168}{131}$ × 100 = 128.

Question 14

Answer D is correct: 50%.

Five countries (UK, US, Can, Pol, Swe) have average monthly text messages in excess of 32 and there are 10 countries in total so $\frac{5}{10}$ × 100 = 50%.

Question 15

Answer E is correct: 4:9.

Any two numbers can be compared by writing them alongside each other separated by a ratio sign (:). There are 200 messages per person per month in the UK and US (81 + 119) and 450 in the other countries (25 + 23 + 26 + 108 + 24 + 31 + 45 + 168). Therefore the ratio is 200:450 which can be simplified to 4:9 by dividing each value by 50.

Question 16

Answer D is correct: €126.00 and $105.00.

The annual average number of text messages in Ireland is 168 × 12 = 2016 × £0.05 = £100.80. The cost in euros is $\frac{100.80}{0.80}$ = €126.00

The annual average number of text messages in the US is 119 × 12 = 1428 × £0.05 = £71.40. The cost in dollars is $\frac{71.40}{0.68}$ = $105.00.

Question 17

Answer B is correct: Between Year 1 and Year 4 the birth rate for women aged 26–35 remained within a margin of 12%.

Between Year 1 and Year 4 the percentage of births for women aged 26–35 ranged from a low of 42% (Year 1) to a high of 54% (Year 2), therefore 54% – 42% = 12% which is within a margin of 12%.

Question 18

Answer C is correct: 250.

In Year 2 women aged 26–35 accounted for 54% of births. If this equated to 750 women giving birth the number of women aged 18–25 giving birth would be $\frac{750}{54}$ × 19 = 263.91 which to the nearest 50 = 250.

Question 19

Answer D is correct: The single highest fall in birth rates during the 4 years was in relation to women aged 18–25.

The birth rate for women aged 18–25 had the highest fall between Year 1 (27%) and Year 2 (19%), an 8% drop.

Question 20

Answer B is correct: 20%.

Add together the percentages over the four years: 13% + 16% + 25% + 25% = 79%. Divide by the number of years to obtain the average percentage, $\frac{79}{4}$ = 19.75%, which is closest to 20%.

Question 21

Answer D is correct: 51.

Obtain the correct data from the table and add the figures together. The classifications less than 71 kilograms are <50, 51–60, and 61–70, so the number of people is 10 + 20 + 21 = 51.

Question 22

Answer C is correct: They are at most 60 kilograms.

Obtain 25% of the total sample of 120 people, i.e. $\frac{120}{100}$ × 25 = 30. Of the choices the only option available to obtain 30 is by adding the first two columns together i.e. <50kg (10) and 51–60kg (20), therefore 25% of the people surveyed 'are at most 60 kilograms'.

Question 23

Answer B is correct: $\frac{1}{3}$.

There are a total of 120 people surveyed and those that weigh in excess of 80 kilograms are: 26 (81–90kg) + 14 (>90kg) = 40 people. 40 as a fraction of 120 is $\frac{40}{120}$ = $\frac{1}{3}$.

Question 24

Answer A is correct: 1:3.

The number of people weighing less than 61 kilograms is 30 and the number weighing 61 kilograms and above is 90. Therefore the ratio is 30:90 which can be simplified to 1:3.

Question 25

Answer E is correct: 30%.

To obtain a percentage divide the number of part-time students by the total number of students and then multiply this by 100, i.e. $\frac{6,037}{19,876} \times 100 = 30.37\%$. You are asked for an approximation, so 30% is correct.

Question 26

Answer A is correct: 2:3.

First obtain the number of students without the science students, $19,876 - 8,241 = 11,635$. The ratio of science students compared to the rest of the students is 8,241:11,635. You are asked for an 'approximation', so round the numbers up or down to the nearest hundred, 8200:11600, which can be simplified to 41:58; round these numbers to 40:60, which can be simplified to 2:3. Alternatively, round the original numbers up or down to the nearest thousand, 8000:12000, which can be simplified to 2:3 by dividing both numbers by 4,000.

Question 27

Answer A is correct: £13m.

Obtain the number of students entitled to a loan which is the total number of students minus the part-time students and science students, i.e. $19,876 - (6,037 + 8,241) = 19,876 - 14,278 = 5,598$. The total cost of student loans is $5,598 \times £2,300 = £12,875,400$, which to the nearest £m is £13m.

Question 28

Answer D is correct: 4,600.

Find out the capacity of the two blocks, i.e. $21 \times 48 = 1,008$ and $38 \times 93 = 3,534$. Add the two figures together, $1,008 + 3,534 = 4,542$; so the best approximation is 4,600.

Question 29

Answer C is correct: 48m².

The area of flooring for one bathroom is 4.2m × 2.4m = 10.08m²; so for four bathrooms is $10.08 \times 4 = 40.32m^2$

One bathroom is $\frac{3}{4}$ of $10.08 = \frac{10.08}{4} \times 3 = 7.56m^2$.

The total floor area is $40.32 + 7.56 = 47.88m^2$, to the nearest whole metre = 48m².

Question 30

Answer E is correct: 112.

The area of a tile measuring 30cm² = $30 \times 30 = 900$cm.

The area of one larger bathroom is 4.2m × 2.4m, or 420cm × 240cm = 100,800cm.

The number of tiles required is $\frac{100800}{900} = 112$.

Question 31

Answer A is correct: $(4200 \times 2400) - (1800 \times 850)$.

The area that requires tiling is the area of the room (4200mm × 2400mm) minus the area of the shower (1800mm × 850mm). Therefore the answer is $(4200 \times 2400) - (1800 \times 850)$.

Question 32

Answer C is correct: £1,122.50.

The price of 500 tiles × £2.75 = £1,375.00 – 12% discount = $\frac{1,375}{100} \times 12$ = £165.00, so £1,375.00 – £165.00 = £1210.00.

500 tiles purchased – 430 used tiles = return of 70 tiles at £1.25 each = £87.50

The floor layer will have paid £1210.00 – £87.50 = £1,122.50.

Question 33

Answer B is correct: 22.

Add the number of values in the column 'number of disputes' and divide by the number of values to obtain the mean. The mean is $\frac{154}{7}$ = 22.

Question 34

Answer C is correct: 25.

The mode is the number in the distribution that has the highest frequency. In this instance the number 25 appears twice and every other number only once.

Question 35

Answer E is correct: 45,840

The range of a distribution is the difference between the highest and lowest values. The highest value is 48,300 and the lowest 2,460, therefore 48,300 – 2,460 = 45,840.

Question 36

Answer A is correct: On average, redundancy had more days lost than any other reason for disputes.

Mental calculations can quickly dismiss all of the options with the exception of Answer A in relation to pay and redundancy. The average days lost per dispute for pay is $\frac{48,300}{52}$ = 928.8. For redundancy it is $\frac{26,125}{24}$ = 1088.5.

Chapter 3
Abstract Reasoning practice subtest 1

Question number	Correct response	Question number	Correct response
1	Set B	34	Neither Set
2	Neither Set	35	Set A
3	Set A	36	Set A
4	Set B	37	Set B
5	Neither Set	38	Neither Set
6	Neither Set	39	Neither Set
7	Neither Set	40	Set A
8	Set B	41	Set A
9	Set A	42	Neither Set
10	Set B	43	Set B
11	Set B	44	Set B
12	Set A	45	Set A
13	Neither Set	46	Set B
14	Set A	47	Set B
15	Neither Set	48	Set A
16	Set B	49	Neither Set
17	Set B	50	Set B
18	Set A	51	Set B
19	Set A	52	Set A
20	Neither Set	53	Set B
21	Set A	54	Set A
22	Set B	55	Set B
23	Neither Set	56	Set A
24	Set A	57	Set B
25	Neither Set	58	Set B
26	Neither Set	59	Neither Set
27	Set A	60	Set A
28	Set B	61	Neither Set
29	Neither Set	62	Set B
30	Set A	63	Set A
31	Set B	64	Neither Set
32	Neither Set	65	Set A
33	Set A		

Questions 1–5

The shapes in Set A all contain three shapes within each other, the outer and inner shapes have solid straight lines, the middle shape has a dotted outline and is curved or part curved. The shapes in Set B also contain three shapes within each other, the outer two shapes have curved or part curved lines and the inner shape has straight lines. The use of black shading and the use of the same shape are distracters. Therefore:

Test shape 1 belongs to Set B as it contains three shapes within each other, the outer two shapes are curved and the inner shape has straight lines.

Test shape 2 belongs to Neither Set as the inner shape would need a solid outline in order to belong to Set A.

Test shape 3 belongs to Set A as it contains three shapes within each other, the outer and inner shapes have solid straight lines, the middle shape has a dotted outline and is curved.

Test shape 4 belongs to Set B as it contains three shapes within each other, the outer two shapes are curved or part curved and the inner shape has straight lines.

Test shape 5 belongs to Neither Set as it contains four shapes within each other.

Questions 6–10

The shapes in Set A all contain at least one white and one grey shaded circle. The shapes in Set B all contain at least one white star and one white square. The use of multiple white, black or grey shapes are all distracters. Therefore:

Test shape 6 belongs to Neither Set as one of the circles would need to be shaded grey in order to belong to Set A.

Test shape 7 belongs to Neither Set as the star would need to be white in order to belong to Set B.

Test shape 8 belongs to Set B as it contains at least one white star and one white square; the circles are incorrect for Set A as one would need to be shaded grey.

Test shape 9 belongs to Set A as it contains at least one white and one grey shaded circle.

Test shape 10 belongs to Set B as it contains at least one white star and one white square; the circles are incorrect for Set A as one would need to be shaded grey.

Questions 11–15

The shapes in Set A all contain two groups of shapes, one group containing two shapes within each other and the other group containing three shapes within each other. The shapes in Set B all contain three shapes within each other, the inner and outer shapes have straight lines and the middle shape has curved lines. The use of curved shapes and straight shapes in Set A; and the use of the same or differing shapes and black or grey shading in both sets are all distracters. Therefore:

Test shape 11 belongs to Set B as it contains three shapes within each other, the inner and outer shapes have straight lines and the middle shape has curved lines.

Test shape 12 belongs to Set A as it contains two groups of shapes, one group containing two shapes within each other and the other group containing three shapes within each other.

Test shape 13 belongs to Neither Set as one of the groups of shapes would need to have three shapes within each other in order to belong to Set A.

Test shape 14 belongs to Set A as it contains two groups of shapes, one group containing two shapes within each other and the other group containing three shapes within each other.

Test shape 15 belongs to Neither Set as the middle and inner shapes would need to be the other way round in order to belong to Set B.

Questions 16–20

The shapes in Set A all contain shapes with straight lines apart from one which has curved lines. The shapes in Set B all contain shapes with curved lines apart from one which has straight lines. The number and size of the shapes and black or grey shading are all distracters. Therefore:

Test shape 16 belongs to Set B as it contains shapes with curved lines apart from one which has straight lines.

Test shape 17 belongs to Set B as it contains shapes with curved lines apart from one which has straight lines.

Test shape 18 belongs to Set A as it contains shapes with straight lines apart from one which has curved lines.

Test shape 19 belongs to Set A as it contains shapes with straight lines apart from one which has curved lines.

Test shape 20 belongs to Neither Set as it contains an equal number of straight and curved line shapes which is not a characteristic of either set.

Questions 21–25

The shapes in Set A are all comprised of four sections. The shapes in Set B are all comprised of six sections. The number of shapes and the holes in the centre of the 'doughnut' shapes are distracters. Therefore:

Test shape 21 belongs to Set A as the shapes are all comprised of four sections.

Test shape 22 belongs to Set B as the shape is comprised of six sections.

Test shape 23 belongs to Neither Set as it contains five sections.

Test shape 24 belongs to Set A as the shape is comprised of four sections.

Test shape 25 belongs to Neither Set as it contains shapes that are comprised of four and six sections and therefore has the attributes of both sets.

Questions 26–30

The shapes in Set A are all made up of four straight lines. The shapes in Set B are all made up of five straight lines. Therefore:

Test shape 26 belongs to Neither Set as it is made up of eight straight lines.

Test shape 27 belongs to Set A as it is made up of four straight lines.

Test shape 28 belongs to Set B as it is made up of five straight lines.

Test shape 29 belongs to Neither Set as it is made up of six straight lines.

Test shape 30 belongs to Set A as it is made up of four straight lines.

Questions 31–35

The shapes in Set A all contain three shapes that overlap creating two overlaps. The shapes in Set B all contain four shapes that overlap creating three overlaps. The use of black and the number of shapes are distracters. Therefore:

Test shape 31 belongs to Set B as it contains four shapes that overlap creating three overlaps.

Test shape 32 belongs to Neither Set as it contains five shapes that overlap creating four overlaps.

Test shape 33 belongs to Set A as it contains three shapes that overlap creating two overlaps.

Test shape 34 belongs to Neither Set as it contains no overlapping shapes.

Test shape 35 belongs to Set A as it contains three shapes that overlap creating two overlaps.

Questions 36–40

The shapes in Set A all contain at least one unique white shape which is not repeated in black. The shapes in Set B all contain at least one unique black shape which is not repeated in white. The use of X's is a distracter. Therefore:

Test shape 36 belongs to Set A as the shape contains one unique white shape.

Test shape 37 belongs to Set B as the shape contains one unique black shape.

Test shape 38 belongs to Neither Set as it does not contain any unique white or black shapes.

Test shape 39 belongs to Neither Set as it contains two black shapes that are the same.

Test shape 40 belongs to Set A as the shape contains one unique white shape.

Questions 41–45

The shapes in Set A all contain at least two shapes the same on a diagonal. The shapes in Set B all contain at least two shapes the same on either the vertical or the horizontal. The use of black or white, the size of the shapes and direction changes, i.e. diagonals, are all distracters. Therefore:

Test shape 41 belongs to Set A as the shape contains two crosses on the diagonal.

Test shape 42 belongs to Neither Set as it contains two hearts on the diagonal and on the horizontal and vertical and therefore has the attributes of both sets.

Test shape 43 belongs to Set B as the shape contains two square shapes on the horizontal.

Test shape 44 belongs to Set B as the shape contains two flag shapes on the vertical.

Test shape 45 belongs to Set A as the shape contains two octagons on the diagonal.

Questions 46–50

The shapes in Set A all contain shapes that have at least one right angle. The shapes in Set B all contain shapes with no right angles. The use of shading, the number of shapes and the use of 3D are all distracters. Therefore:

Test shape 46 belongs to Set B as the shape contains shapes without right angles.

Test shape 47 belongs to Set B as the shape contains shapes without right angles.

Test shape 48 belongs to Set A as the shape contains shapes that all contain at least one right angle.

Test shape 49 belongs to Neither Set as it contains three shapes with at least one right angle and one shape with none and therefore has the attributes of both sets.

Test shape 50 belongs to Set B as the shape contains shapes without right angles.

Questions 51–55

The shapes in Set A cannot be drawn without lifting the pen or pencil off the paper or retracing any line. The shapes in Set B can be drawn without lifting the pen or pencil off the paper or retracing any line. Therefore:

Test shape 51 belongs to Set B as it can be drawn without lifting the pen or pencil off the paper.

Test shape 52 belongs to Set A as it cannot be drawn without lifting the pen or pencil off the paper.

Test shape 53 belongs to Set B as it can be drawn without lifting the pen or pencil off the paper.

Test shape 54 belongs to Set A as it cannot be drawn without lifting the pen or pencil off the paper.

Test shape 55 belongs to Set B as it can be drawn without lifting the pen or pencil off the paper.

Questions 56–60

The shapes in Set A all contain a large shape that is reflected within by a small white shape. The shapes in Set B all contain a large shape that is reflected within by a small black shape. The number of small shapes used and the fact that some small shapes are outside the large shapes are all distracters. Therefore:

Test shape 56 belongs to Set A as the large white heart is reflected within by a small white heart.

Test shape 57 belongs to Set B as the large white doughnut shape is reflected within by a small black doughnut shape.

Test shape 58 belongs to Set B as the large white arrowed square is reflected within by a small black arrowed square.

Test shape 59 belongs to Neither Set as the large white circle contains both a white and black small circle and therefore has the attributes of both sets.

Test shape 60 belongs to Set A as the large white lightning flash is reflected within by a small white lightning flash.

Questions 61–65

The shapes in Set A all contain a shape with a black section which is reflected outside the shape by a white shape. The shapes in Set B all contain a shape with a black section, which is not reflected outside by the white shape. Therefore:

Test shape 61 belongs to Neither Set as it does not contain a shape outside the main shape.

Test shape 62 belongs to Set B as the black section is not reflected in the white shape on the outside of the main shape.

Test shape 63 belongs to Set A as the black section is reflected in the white shape on the outside of the main shape.

Test shape 64 belongs to Neither Set as the black section is reflected as a black shape outside the main shape.

Test shape 65 belongs to Set A as the black section is reflected in the white shape on the outside of the main shape.

Chapter 4
Decision Analysis practice subtest 1

Question number	Correct response
1	Option B
2	Option C
3	Option D
4	Option A
5	Options B & C
6	Option E
7	Option B
8	Option C
9	Option B
10	Option E
11	Option D
12	Option A
13	Option C
14	Options A & E
15	Options B & D
16	Option B
17	Option B
18	Option E
19	Option C
20	Option A
21	Options A & C
22	Option D
23	Option A
24	Option C
25	Option B
26	Option B

Question 1

📷 K, 📄 K, 404, (11 99), ☺

The code combines the words 'sail increase', 'book increase', 'brother', 'happy smile', 'me'

Option B, 'Books on sailing please my brother' is the correct answer as it uses all the codes, with 'sail increase' being used as 'sailing', 'book increase' being used as 'books', 'happy smile' being used as 'please' and 'me' being used as 'my'.

Question 2

(404 606), 404, 606, G, FK, &K, ☺

The code combines the words 'brother cousin', 'brother', 'cousin', 'fight', 'ride increase', 'scooter increase', 'me'

Option C, 'My brother and cousin argue when riding their scooters', is the correct answer as it uses all the codes, with 'brother cousin' being used as 'their', 'fight' being used as 'argue', 'ride increase' being used as 'riding', 'scooter increase' being used as 'scooters' and 'me' being used as 'my'.

Question 3

(505 }), ☺, A, (Ⓟ 🚗)

The code combines the words 'sister skateboard', 'me', 'run', 'police car'

Option D, 'The police car ran over my sister's skateboard', is the correct answer as it uses all the codes, with 'sister skateboard' being used as 'sister's skateboard', 'me' being used as 'my', and 'run' being used as 'ran over'.

Question 4

(am pm), L, ☺ 👪, (J bb Ⴀ 🍽)

The code combines the words 'morning afternoon', 'play', 'me them', 'negative breakfast lunch dinner'

Option A, 'We play all day and forget to eat' is the correct answer as it uses all the codes, with, 'morning afternoon' being used as 'all day', 'me them' being used as 'we' and 'negative breakfast lunch dinner' being used as 'forget to eat'.

Question 5

⬦K, 101, &K, 101, AK

The code combines the words 'bike increase', 'us', 'scooter increase', 'us', 'run increase'

Option B, 'Our bikes are faster than our scooters' and Option C, 'Our scooters aren't as fast as our bikes', are the correct answers as they use all the codes, with 'bike increase' being used as 'bikes', 'us' being used twice as 'our', 'scooter increase' being used as 'scooters', 'run increase' being used as 'faster' in Option B and just as 'fast' in Option C. However, the statements have the same meaning.

Question 6

⬦K, hh, ⬸K, 11, ☺, M 505 ⸙ ⵛ 404

The code combines the words 'bike increase', 'holiday', 'swim increase', 'happy', 'me', 'combine sister mother father brother'

Option E, 'My family enjoy swimming and cycling on holiday', is the correct answer as it uses all the codes, with 'bike increase' being used as 'cycling', 'swim increase' being used as 'swimming', 'happy' being used as 'enjoy', 'me' being used as 'my' and 'combine sister mother father brother' being used as 'family'.

Question 7

707, ⸙, ✸, 808

The code combines the words 'neighbour', 'mother', 'talk', 'doctor'

Option B, 'Mum telephoned the doctor for the lady next door', is the correct answer as it uses all the codes, with 'neighbour' being used as 'lady next door', 'mother' being used as 'mum' and 'talk' being used as 'telephoned'.

Question 8

👽 I, 202, ⸙, 11, 101, ⵛ, M(202 👽 I)

The code combines the words 'enemies opposite', 'we', 'mother', 'happy', 'us', 'lunch', 'combine we enemies opposite'

Option C, 'Our friends are happy when mum lets us have lunch together', is the correct answer as it uses all the codes, with 'enemies opposite' being used as 'friends', 'mother' being used as 'mum', and 'combine we enemies opposite' being used as 'together'.

Question 9

}, 202, ♛ , 707, 00

The code combines the words 'skateboard', 'we', 'them', 'neighbour', 'angry'

Option B, 'Our neighbour was angry and took their skateboard', is the correct answer as it uses all the codes, with 'we' being used as 'our' and 'them' being used as 'their'.

Question 10

33 K, 77 I, 505, E, &, ☺

The code combines the words 'cry increase', 'tall opposite', 'sister', 'fall', 'scooter', 'me'

Option E, 'My small sister fell off her scooter and cried', is the correct answer as it uses all the codes, with 'cry increase' being used as 'cried', 'tall opposite' being used as 'small', 'fall' being used as 'fell', and 'me' being used as 'my'.

Question 11

🚗 K, 202, J 🔁, ☽

The code combines the words 'car increase', 'we', 'negative sleep', 'night'

Option D, 'We had no sleep last night due to traffic', is the correct answer as it uses all the codes, with 'car increase' being used as 'traffic' and 'negative sleep' being used as 'no sleep'.

Question 12

⚓ , 202, 101, 🗑 K, hh, ⏩ K

The code combines the words 'swim', 'we', 'us', 'bucket increase', 'holiday', 'spade increase'

Option A, 'We swim and play with our buckets and spades on holiday', is the correct answer as it uses all the codes, with 'us' being used as 'our', and 'bucket increase' and 'spade increase' being used as 'buckets' and 'spades'.

Question 13

Ⓟ , 🚲 , C K, ⅄, F

The code combines the words 'police', 'bike', ' jump increase', 'lunch', 'ride'

Option C, 'The policeman jumped onto the bike and rode off for lunch', is the correct answer at it uses all the codes, with 'police' being used as 'policeman', 'jump increase' being used as 'jumped', and 'ride' becomes 'rode'.

Question 14

M(404 505), ♦, ☺, ☺, M(K 22 33 00), G

The code combines the words 'combine brother sister', 'mother', 'me', 'me', 'combine increase sad cry angry', 'fight'

Option A, 'Mum gets very emotional when my siblings and I argue', and Option E, 'When I fall out with my siblings mother gets really upset', are the correct answers as they both combine all the codes. Option A uses 'mother' as 'mum' and 'combine increase sad cry angry' as 'very emotional', and 'combine brother sister' as 'siblings', and 'me' and 'me' as 'my' and 'I' respectively, and 'fight' as 'argue'. Option E uses 'fight' as 'fall out' and 'me' and 'me' as 'I' and 'my' respectively, with 'combine brother sister' being used as 'siblings', and 'combine increase sad cry angry' as 'really upset'.

Question 15

Options B and D, 'hot' and 'time', would be the two most useful additions to the codes when attempting to convey the message 'My family are flying off for a holiday in the sun later this year', the word 'hot' being used for 'sun' and the word 'time' being used for 'later'. The other words can be extrapolated from existing codes or are irrelevant.

Question 16

L, tt, 202, ♔, ♦, ☺, M(⚲ ─ ⛝ ─ } ◎)

The code combines the words 'play', 'tomorrow', 'we', 'them', 'talk', 'me', 'combine bike boat car frisbee skateboard ball'

Option B, 'I chat with my friends about which toys we will play with tomorrow' is the correct answer as it uses all the codes, with 'me' being used as both 'I' and 'my', 'them' being used as 'friends', and 'combine bike boat car frisbee skateboard ball' being used as 'toys'.

Question 17

K(99 44), 202, K 11, ☺, M(404 ♦, 505 ϒ)

Option B would be the best way to encode the message 'My family smile and laugh a lot because we are very happy'. This option has the correct codes by using K(99 44) 'increase smile laugh' as 'smile and laugh a lot', K 11 'increase happy' as 'very happy', and M(404 ♦, 505 ϒ) 'combine brother mother sister father' as family.

Question 18

♀, 'Y', 707, 🍽, I 66, 🎤

The code combines the words 'mother', 'father', 'neighbour', 'dinner', 'opposite greedy', 'talk'

Option E, 'The neighbour generously asked mum and dad to dinner', is the correct answer as it uses all the codes, with 'mother' and 'father' being used as 'mum' and 'dad', 'opposite greedy' being used as 'generously', and 'talk' being used as 'asked'.

Question 19

E, 88 ?, 101, I 🚢, ⛴

The code combines the words 'fall', 'small skipping rope', 'us', 'opposite sail', 'boat'

Option C, 'The rope fell off and our boat sank', is the correct answer as it uses all the codes, with 'fall' becoming 'fell', 'small skipping rope' being used as 'rope', and 'opposite sail' being used as 'sank'.

Question 20

K D, ∧, L, 202, nn ww, I, M(☺ 👪)

The code combines the words 'increase fly', 'kite', 'play', 'we', 'now weekend', 'opposite', 'combine me them'

Option A, 'This weekend we are having a kite flying game against each other', is the correct answer as it uses all the codes, with 'now weekend' being 'this weekend', 'increase fly' becoming 'flying', 'play' being used as 'game', 'opposite' becoming 'against', and 'combine me them' being used as 'each other'.

Question 21

Options A and C, 'break' and 'drop', would be the two most useful additions to the codes when attempting to convey the message 'The police said that the paint poured on our car was criminal damage', the word 'break' being used for 'damage' and the word 'drop' being used for 'poured'. The other words can be extrapolated from existing codes or are irrelevant.

Question 22

M(bb Y 🍽), 202, hh, M(♀ 'Y' ☺ 404 505)

The code combines the words 'combine breakfast lunch dinner,' 'we', 'holiday', 'combine mother father me brother sister'

Option D, 'We have all our meals together when on holiday', is the correct answer as it uses all the codes, 'combine breakfast lunch dinner' being used as 'meals' and 'combine mother father me brother sister' being used as 'together'.

Question 23

#, E, 88 🗑, 88 707

The code combines the words 'paint', 'fall', 'small bucket', 'small neighbour'

Option A, 'The child from next door fell over the tin of paint', is the correct answer as it uses all the codes, with 'fall' being used as 'fell over', 'small bucket' being used as 'tin', and 'small neighbour' being interpreted as 'child from next door'.

Question 24

K M(A C H B ⚓), 202, L, M(⚦ Υ ☺ 404 505 606)

The code combines the words 'increase combine run jump climb walk swim', 'we', 'play', 'combine mother father me brother sister cousin'

Option C, 'Our family have very active hobbies', is the correct answer as it uses all the codes, with 'increase combine run jump climb walk swim' being used as 'very active', 'we' being used as 'our', 'play' being used as 'hobbies', and 'combine mother father me brother sister cousin' being used as 'family'.

Question 25

G, 808, ☺, 505, I B, J ⚓

Option B would be the best way to encode the message 'The doctor had to fight to stop my sister from drowning'. This option has the correct codes by using ☺ 'me' as 'my', I B 'opposite walk' as 'stop' and, J 'negative swim' as 'drowning'.

Question 26

✏, Υ, #, nn, 🚗, 55

The code combines the words 'crayon', 'father', 'paint, 'now', 'car', 'jealous'

Option B, 'The paint colour of dad's new car is green', is the correct answer as it uses all the codes, with 'crayon' being used for 'colour', 'now' being used for 'new', and 'jealous' being used for 'green'.

Chapter 5
Verbal Reasoning practice subtest 2

Question number	Correct response	Question number	Correct response
1	C	23	C
2	A	24	B
3	B	25	C
4	A	26	A
5	A	27	B
6	B	28	A
7	C	29	C
8	A	30	C
9	C	31	C
10	B	32	A
11	C	33	B
12	A	34	A
13	A	35	A
14	C	36	C
15	C	37	B
16	A	38	A
17	C	39	C
18	A	40	B
19	C	41	C
20	B	42	B
21	A	43	C
22	C	44	A

Passage I: question 1

C. Can't Tell

This may be the case but cannot be stated with certainty from the information contained in the passage. The passage refers to a trust hospital and it can be inferred that inspections of such hospitals are under the direction of the Healthcare Commission. However, no mention is made of National Health Service hospitals.

Passage I: question 2

A. True

Two examples are provided in the passage to support that statement: 'An audit by the hospital's own trust also found that only 6 out of 10 staff were washing their hands properly, but the trust's board was not informed' and 'The board had also been informed that attendance for mandatory infection control training by staff was acceptable, but in fact it was low'.

Passage I: question 3

B. False

The 22 cases of *C. difficile* are a statement of fact. The passage actually provides information contrary to the statement: 'The hospital has a good record on MRSA and *Clostridium difficile*' and 'These breaches of the Government's hygiene code gave the Commission cause for concern, in spite of the low incidence of infections'.

Passage I: question 4

A. True

The statement is true and can be inferred from the following part of the passage: 'In the endoscopy suite it was not clear whether flexible tubes that are inserted into the body for diagnosis and treatment were ready for sterilisation or had already been decontaminated, even though this had previously been brought to the hospital's attention.' This strongly suggests an external inspection as opposed to an inspection by the trust itself. Where the trust has carried out its own inspections, these are clearly identified in the passage.

Passage II: question 5

A. True

In the last two sentences the passage talks about 'culture shock' and our reaction to another culture resulting in 'fear, which can lead to distrust and hostility'.

Passage II: question 6

B. False

This is a very general statement, and although armed conflicts might more often than not result from cultural differences this may not always be the case. For example, a threat to survival or the actions of egomaniacs may result in conflict.

Passage II: question 7

C. Can't Tell

This might be the case, though to an extent it would tend to contradict the essence of the passage. However, without further information, such as comparative studies with other countries, a true or false answer could not be determined.

Passage II: question 8

A. True

This is essentially the tenet of the passage as it actually states that 'Within those groups we have shared prejudices about other teams …'.

Passage III: question 9

C. Can't Tell

The passage provides two examples – the jatropha tree and algae – from which oil for use with kerosene jet fuel is being tested. It does not state that these are the only sources of alternative oil and further information would be required to clarify this.

Passage III: question 10

B. False

This answer is false as it distinctly states in the passage that this will 'not mean an end to the use of kerosene jet engines, as the amount of jatropha that would be needed to power the entire aviation section can never be produced in a sustainable way'.

Passage III: question 11

C. Can't Tell

In relation to algae the passages states that they 'can be grown in arid regions and virtually anywhere'. However, for the jatropha tree the passage states that this is 'grown on marginal land in India, Mozambique, Malawi and Tanzania'. Although it may be the case that the jatropha tree can be grown in arid regions of the world and virtually anywhere, further information would be required before this can be stated as fact.

Passage III: question 12

A. True

This is true as the passage actually states that 'environmentalists argue that manufacturing biofuels can produce more emissions than they absorb when growing'.

Passage IV: question 13

A. True

This statement can be accepted as accurate as there is no mention in the passage of universities relaxing their entry criteria and there is no doubt that the additional 35,000 students had been accepted in defiance of the 13,000 government cap.

Passage IV: question 14

C. Can't Tell

Although it might be assumed that the university population is still mainly students under 25, this is not made explicit in the passage. The only real reference made is to the fact that 'There were an additional 60,000 applications for places in the current year, comprising a 10% increase in students overall but a 19.5% rise among students over 25 years of age'. However, this does not provide details of what numbers the increases were based on.

Passage IV: question 15

C. Can't Tell

Although redundancy and job insecurity may be a factor that has increased the number of over-25s going to university, there are no reasons for the increase contained in the passage. Further information would be required before a 'true' or 'false' answer could be given.

Passage IV: question 16

A. True

This can be accepted from the statement that, 'the number of overseas students doubling in the past 10 years'. Next to the government, they are the biggest source of the universities' funding.

Passage V: question 17

C. Can't Tell

The passage actually states that cars operate more efficiently above 30mph. However, there is no mention of lorries performing more efficiently above this speed and there is also no information about a maximum speed whereby efficiency decreases; this may be less than 70mph.

Passage V: question 18

A. True

The passage states, 'Also there is an understandable deep-rooted concern about Big Brother!' and implicit in this is the fact that speed limiters *might* lead to a greater infringement of civil liberties.

Passage V: question 19

C. Can't Tell

Although speed limiters are already fitted to the engines of some lorries, there is no information about this in the passage. Therefore further information about this, together with comparative technical details concerning the pros and cons of existing and proposed speed limiters, would be required.

Passage V: question 20

B. False

The passage states that 'The Commission for Integrated Transport and the Motorists' Forum claim that accidents involving injuries could be cut by 12 per cent' or more where it was mandatory that speed limiters were fitted to vehicles. This statement envisages that there would be a reduction in accidents involving injury that would undoubtedly include vehicles driven by newly qualified drivers.

Passage VI: question 21

A. True

The passage actually states that '23 per cent of men and 15 per cent of women drink more than twice the government's recommended daily limit'. The passage also states that heavy drinkers are at an increased risk of permanent brain damage.

Passage VI: question 22

C. Can't Tell

The passage states that heavy drinkers are at an increased risk of engaging in unprotected sex. However, those who drink excessively only account for less than one quarter of the population. In relation to unprotected sex, no figures are provided for either drinkers or other groups that do not drink excessively, so further information would be required before a true or false answer could be made.

Passage VI: question 23

C. Can't Tell

The passage does state, 'Alcohol-related brain damage is an increasing burden on the NHS, and patients who do not die early with the condition…'. However, no comparative figures are provided with other illnesses, diseases, or demographic factors that may be relevant. Further information would be required to support this statement.

Passage VI: question 24

B. False

The passage says that '23 per cent of men and 15 per cent of women drink more than twice the government's recommended daily limit'. If 15 per cent of women were heavy drinkers, for men to be twice as likely to be heavy drinkers the figure would need to be 30 per cent of men, i.e. 15 × 2, and not 23 per cent as given.

Passage VII: question 25

C. Can't Tell

In relation to 'bad parenting' the passage states, 'There are the possible positive and negative effects of…good and bad parenting.' It does not elaborate in relation to health matters of children in later life and further information would be required.

Passage VII: question 26

A. True

This is specifically stated in the passage: ' …more frequent occurrence of delirium with infection at the extremes of the age spectrum.'

Passage VII: question 27

B. False

The passage states, 'Early upbringing will also influence health in later life. There are the possible positive and negative effects of…parental smoking and alcohol use…' The question states that, 'Parental smoking or alcohol abuse has no adverse effect…' This is incorrect as it may have an adverse effect.

Passage VII: question 28

A. True

The passage clearly states, 'Generally, older people see their health as functioning even in the presence of chronic disease while young people see health more as fitness.'

Passage VIII: question 29

C. Can't Tell

In relation to offenders undertaking community service the passage states that 'such sentences may result in fewer people being sent to prison'; note the word 'may'. Further information would be required to answer this question either as true or false.

Passage VIII: question 30

C. Can't Tell

Although the fact that 'the government consider that any shame felt by offenders is the shame ... of having committed an offence', clearly this doesn't mean that all offenders feel this shame; neither can we assume that none of these offenders feel ashamed. We have no way of knowing who feels ashamed and who does not, so the answer must be Can't Tell.

Passage VIII: question 31

C. Can't Tell

The final sentence of the passage covers this statement, i.e. 'the Probation Service has highlighted the fact that there have been a number of attacks on offenders undertaking community service and that the use of bright orange bibs is almost certain to increase the risk'. Although the Probation Service consider an increase in attacks highly likely, as yet there is no evidence to substantiate this and further information would be required.

Passage VIII: question 32

A. True

This is actually stated within the passage: '…putting offenders in stocks; that it is about shaming people'.

Passage IX: question 33

B. False

This is obviously false as the 200 pigs would still be producing 100 tons of carbon equivalent each year irrespective of the tax.

Passage IX: question 34

A. True

The last line of the passage states that cattle and pig farms going out of business would have 'a knock-on effect of wide-scale closures of food outlets across the country'. This indicates that there would be a shortage of pig and cattle products if the farms closed, and this shortage would mean many food outlets had nothing to sell.

Passage IX: question 35

A. True

This is true, as clearly stated in the second sentence of the passage: 'They consider this an environmental issue and say that farmers should be charged for rising levels of methane and other polluting nitrous gases emitted by farm animals.'

Passage IX: question 36

C. Can't Tell

Although farm animals' belching and flatulence do have a carbon footprint it is not clear from the passage how 'significant' this actually is. It is difficult to assess what 100 tons of carbon equivalent is as there are no comparative measures.

Passage X: question 37

B. False

The passage states, '11 per cent of offenders released from prison are back in prison after two years from being released. During the two-year period overall nearly half (46 per cent) of offenders started another prison sentence at some point.' This means that of the 46 per cent a number started another prison sentence after two years from being released.

Passage X: question 38

A. True

The final sentence states '…compared with 42 per cent for the average JSA claimant.'

Passage X: question 39

C. Can't Tell

The passage states: '11 per cent of offenders released from prison are back in prison after two years from being released.' From this it can be deduced that 89% are not back in prison after two years from being released. However, they may not have been apprehended for offences committed and therefore further information would be required.

Passage X: question 40

B. False

The passage states, 'On average, offenders leaving prison spent 48 per cent of the next two years on out-of-work benefits.' The 47 per cent relates to offenders on out-of-work benefits after two years of their release from prison.

Passage XI: question 41

C. Can't Tell

Although the passage states, 'As might be expected, the vast majority of people who have both low incomes and live in very energy-inefficient housing are in fuel poverty,' specific measures for increasing energy efficiency such as loft insulation and double-glazing are not mentioned and therefore further information would be required.

Passage XI: question 42

B. False

The passage states, 'It is thus a measure which compares income with what the fuel costs "should be" rather than what they actually are.'

Passage XI: question 43

C. Can't Tell

This is not specifically referred to in the passage. There is no mention in the statement in relation to people in rural areas on 'low income' and further information would be required.

Passage XI: question 44

A. True

The passage actually states, '…two of the low-income groups with high rates of fuel poverty are single-person households of working age…'

Chapter 6
Quantitative Reasoning practice subtest 2

Question number	Correct response	Question number	Correct response
1	C	19	C
2	E	20	A
3	D	21	A
4	B	22	D
5	C	23	A
6	A	24	D
7	B	25	B
8	E	26	D
9	C	27	E
10	B	28	C
11	A	29	B
12	D	30	C
13	D	31	D
14	B	32	D
15	E	33	E
16	E	34	D
17	D	35	D
18	B	36	B

Question 1

Answer C is correct: £382.50.

The cost of the theatre company per session is £37.50, so 12 sessions cost £37.50 × 12 = £450.00. 85% of £450 = $\frac{450}{100}$ × 85 = £382.50.

Question 2

Answer E is correct: £35.50.

The range of a distribution is the difference between the highest and lowest values. The highest value is £37.50 and the lowest value of £2.00, therefore the range is £37.50 − £2.00 = £35.50.

Question 3

Answer D is correct: 28%.

In relation to shop training the user cost is £32.50 and the charity cost is £23.25. The 'profit' made is £32.50 − £23.25 = £9.25. The 'profit' as a percentage of user cost is $\frac{9.25}{32.50} \times 100 = 28\%$.

Question 4

Answer B is correct: £13.80.

Add the costs for each activity: theatre company £37.50 + rural craft (×2) £15.50 + badminton £2.50 + yoga £4.00 = £59.50. Personal budget of £78.20 − £59.50 = £18.70. The amount of additional money they would need to attend shop training is the cost of the training £32.50 − £18.70 = £13.80.

Question 5

Answer C is correct: 180.10 minutes.

Find the mean running time by summing the values of the top ten women runners and dividing by the number of values. Convert the running times to minutes. First sum the value of the hours = 26, convert to minutes, 26 × 60 = 1,560 minutes. Then sum the value of the minutes = 241 minutes. Add these together, so 1,560 + 241 = 1,801 minutes. Divide by the number of values, $\frac{1,801}{10}$ = 180.10 minutes.

Question 6

Answer A is correct: 38 minutes.

The mode is the number in the distribution that has the highest frequency. For the men's half marathon the time 2 hours 48 minutes is the only one to appear more than once. For the women's half marathon the time 3 hours 2 minutes is the only one to appear more than once. Therefore the difference between the mode running times for the men's and women's half marathon is 3 hours 2 minutes − 2 hours 48 minutes = 14 minutes.

Question 7

Answer B is correct: 2 hours 44 minutes.

To find the median of a set of values where there is an even number add the two middle values together and divide by 2. The middle two running times are 2 hours 42 minutes and 2 hours 46 minutes, so the median is $\frac{2.42 + 2.46}{2}$ = 2 hours 44 minutes.

Question 8

Answer E is correct: 55%

In the men's half marathon 4 runners had times less than 2 hours 46 minutes. In the women's half marathon 7 runners had times less than 3 hours 5 minutes. Therefore 4 + 7 = 11 runners out of the 20 who reached the qualifying time. 11 as a percentage of 20 = $\frac{11}{20}$ × 100 = 55%.

Question 9

Answer C is correct: 41%.

Obtain the percentage by writing the first number as a fraction of the second and multiplying by 100. 31 clubs have a turnover in excess of £8m (23 + 8) and there are 75 clubs in total, so $\frac{31}{75}$ × 100 = 41.33%, rounded down to 41%.

Question 10

Answer B is correct: A$8,500,000.

The minimum turnover in this group is £4.1m. To convert this to Australian dollars multiply by the conversion rate, £4.1m × A$2.10 = A$8,610,000, which to the nearest A$500,000 is A$8,500,000.

Question 11

Answer A is correct: 8.

Obtain 60% of 900 which is $\frac{900}{100}$ × 60 = 540, and this leaves 900 − 540 = 360 employees. These 360 are spread pro rata across 44 clubs, therefore each of these clubs employs $\frac{360}{44}$ = 8.18 staff, which to the nearest whole number is 8.

Question 12

Answer D is correct: 1:4.

Any two numbers can be compared by writing them alongside each other separated by a ratio (:) sign. There are 15 clubs with a turnover between £6.1m and £10m (7 + 8) and there are 60 other clubs (75 − 15). Therefore the ratio is 15:60, which can be simplified to 1:4.

Question 13

Answer D is correct: £87.75.

To apply one coat: 7.5m × 2.75m × 2 = 41.25, rounded to 42 square metres + 3.5m × 2.75m = 9.625, rounded to 10 square metres = 52 square metres. One 5 litre tin of paint covers 12 square metres, therefore the amount of paint required is 52 square metres divided by 12 square metres = 4.3 tins of paint. Double this for two coats of paint, 4.3 × 2 = 8.6 tins of paint. Therefore 9 tins will be required at a total cost of 9 × £9.75 = £87.75.

Question 14

Answer B is correct: 4.

The width of the wall is 3.5m (350cm) and the width of the paper is 55cm therefore $\frac{350}{55}$ = 6.36, therefore 7 widths of wallpaper will be required. The height of the wall is 2.75m, so 2.75m × 7 = 19.25m is the total length of wallpaper needed. Each roll of wallpaper is 5m long, therefore $\frac{19.25}{5}$ = 3.85 rolls of wallpaper are required, which rounded to the highest whole number is 4.

Question 15

Answer E is correct: 35m.

For the side wall without the door, the width of the wall is 3.5m (350cm) the width of the paper is 55cm, so $\frac{350}{55}$ = 6.36, therefore 7 widths of wallpaper will be required. The height of the wall is 2.75m, so 2.75m × 7 = 19.25m is the total length of wallpaper needed for that wall.

For the side wall with the door, initially assume there is no door so the length of wallpaper is the same as for the other wall at 19.25m. Calculate the depth of the door that accounts for two 55cm widths of wallpaper: 1.75 × 2 = 3.5. Deduct this from the total length: 19.25m – 3.5m = 15.75m. Add these two figures together to arrive at total length of wallpaper for both side walls: 19.25 + 15.75 = 35m.

Question 16

Answer D is correct: £520.00.

Cost of paint: £9.75 × 7 = £68.25 – 20% ($\frac{68.25}{100}$ × 20 = 13.65) = £54.60.

Cost of wallpaper: £2.65 × 8 = £21.20 – 20% ($\frac{21.20}{100}$ × 20 = 4.24) = £16.96.

Labour costs: £18.50 × 20 = £370.00 + VAT ($\frac{370}{100}$ × 20 = 74) = £444.00.

The total cost of the job is £54.60 + £16.96 + £444.00 = £515.56, to the nearest £10.00 is £520.00.

Question 17

Answer D is correct: 3,100.

Detected crime resulting in a charge or court summons is 49% of 1.37m, i.e. $\frac{1,370,000}{100} \times 49 = 671,300$.

Detected crime resulting in spot fines, warnings and police cautions is 207,500 + 104,000 + 362,900 = 674,400.

Therefore 674,400 – 671,300 = 3,100 more people were dealt with by spot fines, warnings or cautions than were dealt with by a charge or court summons.

Question 18

Answer B is correct: 15.15%.

There were 207,500 spot fines. Calculate 1% of total crime of 1.37m = $\frac{1,370,000}{100} = 13,700$. So the percentage of spot fines is $\frac{207,500}{13,700} = 15.15\%$.

Question 19

Answer C is correct: 2:7.

Any two numbers can be compared by writing them alongside each other separated by a ratio (:) sign. There were 104,000 cannabis warnings and 362,900 police cautions. The ratio is 104,000:362,900 – for an approximate ratio this can be rounded to 100,000:350,000, which can be simplified to 100:350 and then to 2:7.

Question 20

Answer A is correct: 503,797.

Number of detected crimes in 10 years will increase by: $\frac{1,370,000}{100} \times 18 = 246,600$ and 1,370,000 + 246,600 = 1,616,600.

Last year spot fines, warnings and cautions accounted for 51% of detected crime: $\frac{1,370,000}{100} \times 51 = 698,700$.

Percentage relating to police cautions is $\frac{362,900}{698,700} \times 100 = 51.94\%$.

In 10 years' time 40% of detected crime results in a charge or court summons, $\frac{1,616,600}{100} \times 40 = 646,640$ people, therefore spot fines, warnings and cautions account for 1,616,600 – 646,640 = 969,960.

If police cautions still account for 51.94%, the number of people cautioned will be $\frac{969,960}{100} \times 51.94 = 503,797$.

Question 21

Answer A is correct: $17\frac{3}{4}$ hours.

The flight time from the UK to New Zealand via China is $11\frac{1}{4} + 16 = 27\frac{1}{4}$ hours. Adding a stopover of 4 days (96 hours) gives $27\frac{1}{4} + 96 = 123\frac{1}{4}$ hours.

The flight time from the UK to Australia via Dubai is $7\frac{1}{2} + 14 = 21\frac{1}{2}$ hours. Adding a stopover of $3\frac{1}{2}$ days (84 hours) gives $21\frac{1}{2} + 84 = 105\frac{1}{2}$ hours.

The difference in time is $123\frac{1}{4} - 105\frac{1}{2} = 17\frac{3}{4}$ hours.

Question 22

Answer D is correct: £4,908.75.

A single fare: UK to China = $6,250 \times £0.15 = £937.50$. China to New Zealand = $9,750 \times £0.20 = £1,950.00$. Cost of single fare to New Zealand via China = £937.50 + £1,950 = £2,887.50.

Cost of return fare is $£2,887.50 \times 2 = £5,775.00$, –15%. Reduction of 15% is $\frac{5,775}{100} \times 15 = £866.25$. Therefore total cost = £5,775.00 – £866.25 = £4,908.75.

Question 23

Answer A is correct: 2 minutes.

Dubai flight: $7\frac{1}{2}$ hours (flying time) + 4 hours (GMT +4) + 1 hour 12 minutes delay = 12 hours 42 minutes. Dubai time = 10.00 hours + 12 hours 42 minutes = 22.42 hours Monday.

Hawaii flight: 17 hours (flying time) – 10 hours (GMT –10) + 5 hours 20 minutes = 12 hours 20 minutes. Hawaii time = 10.00 + 12 hours 20 minutes = 22.40 hours Monday.

Question 24

Answer D is correct: $26\frac{1}{2}$ hours.

The distance to Australia with a stopover in Fiji is 12,800 + 2,300 = 15,100 miles. To calculate the time for the Boeing 787 divide the number of miles by the average speed i.e. $\frac{15,100}{570} = 26.49$ hours, which to the nearest half hour is 26.5 or $26\frac{1}{2}$.

Question 25

Answer B is correct: 61,782.

1981 the population was 56,352 and in 2001 was 59,009.

The percentage increase between 1981 and 2001 is 59,009 − 56,352 = 2,657, then $\frac{2,657}{56,352} \times 100$ = 4.7%.

The population in 2021 would be 59,009 + 4.7% = $\frac{59,009}{100} \times 4.7$ = 2,773; 59,009 + 2,773 = 61,782.

Question 26

Answer D is correct: In the 20th century the percentage growth rate in Northern Ireland has exceeded that in Scotland.

The percentage growth rate in Northern Ireland; 1,675 (2001) − 1,237 (1901) = 438; $\frac{438}{1,237} \times 100 = 35.4\%$.

The growth rate in Scotland; 5,123 (2001) − 4,479 (1901) = 644; $\frac{644}{4,479} \times 100 = 14.4\%$.

The percentage growth rate in Northern Ireland far exceeded that in Scotland.

Question 27

Answer E is correct: $\frac{1}{8}$

Population in Scotland in 1941 was 5,160 and in England and Wales was 41,748.

Expressed as a fraction, $\frac{5,160}{41,748}$, which to approximate can be rounded down to $\frac{5,000}{40,000}$, divide both by 5,000 = $\frac{1}{8}$.

Question 28

Answer C is correct: 19,178.

1951 >50 population was 25%; 1991 >50 population was 31%; an increase of 6% in four decades.

Between 1991 and 2001 (one decade) the percentage increase would be: $\frac{6\%}{4}$ = 1.5%, so that 31% + 1.5% = 32.5% of the UK population would be over 50.

32.5% of the 2001 UK population is $\frac{59,009}{100} \times 32.5$ = 19,177.992 = 19,178.

Question 29

Answer B is correct: 1 hour 40 minutes.

60 minutes/30 mph × 20 miles = 40 minutes.

60 minutes/60 mph × 40 miles = 40 minutes.

60 minutes/30 mph × 10 miles = 20 minutes.

Total time = 40 + 40 + 20 = 1 hour 40 minutes.

Question 30

Answer C is correct: 210.94 miles.

Journey time 3 hours = 180 minutes.

$\frac{1}{4}$ of journey is $\frac{180}{4}$ = 45 minutes. $\frac{90}{60}$ × 45 = 67.5 kilometres.

$\frac{3}{4}$ of journey is $\frac{180}{4}$ × 3 = 135 minutes. $\frac{120}{60}$ × 135 = 270 kilometres.

Total kilometres: 67.5 + 270 = 337.5 kilometres. Convert to miles: $\frac{337.5}{1.6}$ = 210.94 miles.

Question 31

Answer D is correct: 718.75 kilometres.

Total fuel used = 75 + $\frac{2}{3}$ of 75 = 125 litres. Kilometres travelled = 125 × 5.75 = 718.75 kilometres.

Question 32

Answer D is correct: 12 laps.

Distance travelled: 80 mph for 3 minutes = $\frac{80}{60}$ × 3 = 4 miles; 110 mph for 12 minutes = $\frac{110}{60}$ × 12 = 22 miles; 140 mph for 15 minutes = $\frac{140}{60}$ × 15 = 35 miles. Total distance 4 + 22 + 35 = 61 miles.

No of laps completed: $\frac{61}{5}$ = 12.2, therefore 12 full laps completed.

Question 33

Answer E is correct: 1,150.

If $\frac{1}{3}$ of women's deaths = 575 then the men's deaths account for $\frac{2}{3}$, which is 575 × 2 = 1,150.

Question 34

Answer A is correct: Between 1985 and 2004 the average death rate for people over 70 exceeded the average death rate for people 31 to 50 by over 44%.

Over 70: 61% + 54% + 57% + 60% = 232. $\frac{232}{4}$ = 58%.

31–50: 10% + 15%+ 16% + 14% = 55. $\frac{55}{4}$ = 13.75%.

Difference is 58% – 13.75% = 44.25%, so deaths for people over 70 did exceed the average death rate of people aged 31–50 by over 44%.

Question 35

Answer D is correct: 4:1

Between 2000 and 2004, 60% of deaths are of those aged over 70; 14% are of those aged 31–50. The ratio is therefore 60:14, which is approximately 60:15 or 4:1.

Question 36

Answer B is correct: The largest percentage change in the death rate has occurred in people aged over 70.

The largest percentage change in the death rate in any group is the 7 percentage point fall for the over-70 group between 1985–89 and 1990–94.

Chapter 7
Abstract Reasoning practice subtest 2

Question number	Correct response	Question number	Correct response
1	Neither Set	34	Set A
2	Set A	35	Set A
3	Set A	36	Set B
4	Neither Set	37	Neither Set
5	Set B	38	Set A
6	Neither Set	39	Set B
7	Set A	40	Set A
8	Neither Set	41	Neither Set
9	Set B	42	Set A
10	Set B	43	Neither Set
11	Neither Set	44	Set B
12	Set B	45	Set A
13	Set B	46	Set B
14	Set A	47	Neither Set
15	Set A	48	Set A
16	Neither Set	49	Set B
17	Set B	50	Neither Set
18	Neither Set	51	Set B
19	Neither Set	52	Neither Set
20	Set A	53	Neither Set
21	Set B	54	Set A
22	Neither Set	55	Set B
23	Set B	56	Neither Set
24	Set A	57	Neither Set
25	Neither Set	58	Set B
26	Set A	59	Neither Set
27	Set A	60	Set A
28	Neither Set	61	Set A
29	Set B	62	Set A
30	Set B	63	Set B
31	Neither Set	64	Neither Set
32	Neither Set	65	Set A
33	Set B		

Questions 1–5

The spots on the dominoes in Set A add up to an even number; each domino has an odd number of spots; the left-hand domino has the highest value at the top and the right hand domino has the highest value at the bottom. The spots on the dominoes in Set B add up to an odd number; the left-hand domino adds up to an odd number; the right-hand domino adds up to an even number and the highest value is at the bottom of both dominoes. Therefore:

Test shape 1 belongs to Neither Set as both dominoes are an even number and this does not fit the characteristics of either set.

Test shape 2 belongs to Set A as the spots on the dominoes add up to an even number; each domino has an odd number of spots; the left-hand domino has the highest value at the top and the right-hand domino has the highest value at the bottom.

Test shape 3 belongs to Set A as the spots on the dominoes add up to an even number; each domino has an odd number of spots; the left-hand domino has the highest value at the top and the right-hand domino has the highest value at the bottom.

Test shape 4 belongs to Neither Set as the values add up to an even number as in Set A, but the highest values on the two dominoes are at the bottom left and top right, which is the reverse of the requirement for Set A.

Test shape 5 belongs to Set B as the spots on the dominoes add up to an odd number; the left-hand domino adds up to an odd number; the right-hand domino adds up to an even number and the highest value is at the bottom of both dominoes.

Questions 6–10

The shapes in Set A add up to an even number and half of the shapes are black. The shapes in Set B add up to an odd number and all but one are white. The use of different shading in Set B is a distracter as are items that contain the same shape. Therefore:

Test shape 6 belongs to Neither Set as the shapes add up to an odd number but more than one is black.

Test shape 7 belongs to Set A as the shapes add up to an even number and half are black.

Test shape 8 belongs to Neither Set since even though the shapes add up to an odd number, there are two shapes shaded instead of just one.

Test shape 9 belongs to Set B as the shapes add up to an odd number and all but one are white.

Test shape 10 belongs to Set B as the shapes add up to an odd number and all but one are white.

Questions 11–15

The two clock shapes in Set A have clockwise angles from the large hand to the small hand that add up to either 90 or 150 degrees (15 minutes or 25 minutes). The two clock shapes in Set B have clockwise angles from the large hand to the small hand that add up to 270 degrees (45 minutes). Therefore:

Test shape 11 belongs to Neither Set as the two clock shapes have angles that add up to 120 degrees (20 minutes).

Test shape 12 belongs to Set B as the two clock shapes have angles that add up to 270 degrees (45 minutes).

Test shape 13 belongs to Set B as the two clock shapes have angles that add up to 270 degrees (45 minutes).

Test shape 14 belongs to Set A as the two clock shapes have angles that add up to 150 degrees (25 minutes).

Test shape 15 belongs to Set A as the two clock shapes have angles that add up to 90 degrees (15 minutes).

Questions 16–20

The shapes in Set A all have four enclosed areas; if a shape with a curved side overlaps one with a straight side then the overlap is grey. The shapes in Set B all have five enclosed areas; if shapes with straight sides overlap then the remainder of the shape is black. Therefore:

Test shape 16 belongs to Neither Set as the overlap area would need to be grey for Set A and there are insufficient enclosed areas for Set B.

Test shape 17 belongs to Set B as there are five enclosed areas and no overlapping straight sided shapes.

Test shape 18 belongs to Neither Set as the remainder of the overlapping straight sided shapes should have been black in order to belong to Set B.

Test shape 19 belongs to Neither Set as the overlap between the square and the circle should have been grey in order to belong to Set A.

Test shape 20 belongs to Set A as there are four enclosed areas and the overlap between a curved and a straight side is shaded grey.

Questions 21–25

The shapes in Set A have two shapes that create one overlap and the bottom right-hand corner is always blank. The shapes in Set B have three shapes that create two overlaps and the top left-hand corner is always blank. The number of shapes and shading are distracters. Therefore:

Test shape 21 belongs to Set B as the Test shape has three shapes that create two overlaps and the top left-hand corner is blank.

Test shape 22 belongs to Neither Set as the Test shape has four shapes that create three overlaps which is not a requirement for either set.

Test shape 23 belongs to Set B as the Test shape has three shapes that create two overlaps and the top left-hand corner is blank.

Test shape 24 belongs to Set A as the Test shape has two shapes that create one overlap and the bottom right-hand corner is blank.

Test shape 25 belongs to Neither Set as it does not contain any overlapping shapes and there are no blank corners.

Questions 26–30

The shapes in Set A are all made up of grids which contain 40 black squares and the remaining 24 squares have 2 grey squares vertically adjacent. The shapes in Set B are all made up of grids which contain 32 black squares and the remaining 32 squares have 3 grey squares horizontally adjacent. Therefore:

Test shape 26 belongs to Set A as the grid contains 40 black squares and 2 grey squares vertically adjacent.

Test shape 27 belongs to Set A as the grid contains 40 black squares and 2 grey squares vertically adjacent.

Test shape 28 belongs to Neither Set as the grid only contains 24 black squares which is an invalid requirement.

Test shape 29 belongs to Set B as the grid contains 32 black squares and 3 grey squares horizontally adjacent.

Test shape 30 belongs to Set B as the grid contains 32 black squares and 3 grey squares horizontally adjacent.

Questions 31–35

The shapes in Set A all contain a small, medium and large shape; counting double for shaded shapes, the number of lines used to create the shapes equals 17. The shapes in Set B all contain a large grey shape and two small white shapes; counting double for the small white shapes, the number of lines used to create the shapes equals 28. Therefore:

Test shape 31 belongs to Neither Set as it contains shapes that would require 21 lines if the shaded shape is doubled as in Set A, and it does not fit the characteristics of Set B.

Test shape 32 belongs to Neither Set as it contains three shapes that are the same size, which is not a requirement for either Set.

Test shape 33 belongs to Set B as it contains a large grey shape and two small white shapes; counting double for the small white shapes, the number of lines used to create the shapes equals 28.

Test shape 34 belongs to Set A as it contains a small, medium and large shape; counting double for the shaded shape, the number of lines used to create the shapes equals 17.

Test shape 35 belongs to Set A as it contains a small, medium and large shape; counting double for the shaded shape the number of lines used to create the shapes equals 17.

Questions 36–40

The shapes in Set A all contain the same number of hearts as there are right angles in the straight-sided shapes. The shapes in Set B all contain one more circular shape than the number of straight-sided shapes without right angles. The use of black or white hearts or circles are distracters. Therefore:

Test shape 36 belongs to Set B as it contains one more circular shape than the number of straight-sided shapes without right angles.

Test shape 37 belongs to Neither Set as it does not contain the correct number of hearts in relation to the number of right angles.

Test shape 38 belongs to Set A as it contains the same number of hearts as there are right angles in the straight-sided shapes.

Test shape 39 belongs to Set B as it contains one more circular shape than the number of straight sided shapes without right angles.

Test shape 40 belongs to Set A as it contains the same number of hearts as there are right angles in the straight-sided shape.

Questions 41–45

The shapes in Set A contain eight shapes (ignoring the centre shape) which rotate clockwise in the same order in each square but the rotation does not always follow from square to square, the same shapes are always white, black, grey and striped; in addition the centre shape is always the same as the top right-hand shape but always has the colour of the top left-hand shape. The shapes in Set B contain eight shapes (ignoring the centre shape) which rotate clockwise in the same order in each square and the rotations follow clockwise starting from left to right across each row; in addition, the centre circle is grey when two circles are on the diagonal, black when two circles are on the horizontal and white when two circles are on the vertical. Therefore:

Test shape 41 belongs to Neither Set as the centre shape is shaded rather than white.

Test shape 42 belongs to Set A as the shapes rotate clockwise in the same order and the centre shape is a star which is striped.

Test shape 43 belongs to Neither Set as it contains three circular shapes which is not a characteristic of either Set A or Set B.

Test shape 44 belongs to Set B as the shapes rotate clockwise in the same order and it would be the next square in the sequence if the rotation continued; in addition the centre circle is grey as the circles are on a diagonal.

Test shape 45 belongs to Set A as the shapes rotate clockwise in the same order and the centre shape is a cross which is white.

Questions 46–50

The shapes in Set A all join together to make the same size solid circle. The shapes in Set B all join together to make the same size solid square. The black shading is irrelevant.

Test shape 46 belongs to Set B as the shapes would form the same size solid square.

Test shape 47 belongs to Neither Set as the shapes would join together to form a solid triangle.

Test shape 48 belongs to Set A as the shapes would form the same size solid circle.

Test shape 49 belongs to Set B as the shapes would form the same size solid square.

Test shape 50 belongs to Neither Set as the shapes would form either a cross or a square with a hole in the centre which would be incorrect for Set B.

Questions 51–55

The shapes in Set A all contain arrows and hearts; if at least two arrows point up then the lower heart is grey; if at least two arrows point down then the upper heart is grey; arrows can be either black or white and two hearts are always white, and one is always grey. The shapes in Set B all contain arrows and hearts; if at least two arrows point left then the lower heart is white; if at least two arrows point right then the upper heart is white; arrows can be either black or white, and two hearts are always grey, and one is always white. Therefore:

Test shape 51 belongs to Set B as the two arrows point right and the white heart is uppermost.

Test shape 52 belongs to Neither Set as the arrows and hearts are the wrong shades for either Set.

Test shape 53 belongs to Neither Set as the arrows and hearts are the wrong shades for either Set.

Test shape 54 belongs to Set A as at least two arrows point up and the grey heart is below the two white hearts.

Test shape 55 belongs to Set B as at least two arrows point left and the white heart is below the two grey hearts.

Questions 56–60

The shapes in Set A contain a single grey diamond, but where there are two diamonds the right-hand diamond is black, there are three different white shapes; if other shapes are present, they are grey circles. The shapes in Set B contain a single white diamond, but where there are two diamonds the diamond closer to the top is grey; there are two white shapes with an additional black shape which matches one of the two; if other shapes are present, they are black circles. Therefore:

Test shape 56 belongs to Neither Set as the uppermost diamond would need to be grey for the shape to belong to Set B.

Test shape 57 belongs to Neither Set as the diamond to the left would need to be grey for the shape to belong to Set A.

Test shape 58 belongs to Set B as it contains a grey diamond above a white diamond and two white shapes with one repeated in black.

Test shape 59 belongs to Neither Set as the lower diamond would need to be white in order to belong to Set B.

Test shape 60 belongs to Set A as it contains a single grey diamond; three different white shapes and the additional shapes are grey circles.

Questions 61–65

The shapes in Set A contain a chevron that points to the left if two or more irregular shapes are present; otherwise the arrow points right; if a diamond is present then the arrow is black. The shapes in Set B contain a chevron which points right if two or more irregular shapes are present; otherwise the arrow points left; if a heart is present then the arrow is black.

Test shape 61 belongs to Set A as it contains four irregular shapes with a white chevron pointing left as no diamond is present.

Test shape 62 belongs to Set A as it contains no irregular shapes and a black chevron pointing right as a diamond is present.

Test shape 63 belongs to Set B as it contains three irregular shapes with a black chevron pointing right as a triangle is present.

Test shape 64 belongs to Neither Set as it contains two irregular shapes with a diamond but the chevron is pointing right instead of left.

Test shape 65 belongs to Set A as it contains no irregular shapes and a white chevron pointing right as no diamond is present.

Chapter 8
Decision Analysis practice subtest 2

Question number	Correct response
1	A
2	B
3	E
4	C
5	C
6	D
7	A
8	E
9	B & C
10	C
11	C
12	B
13	D
14	E
15	A
16	B
17	C
18	D
19	E
20	E
21	D
22	A
23	A & D
24	B
25	A & E
26	C

Question 1

312, 213 Z, œ, U, 123, Ω

The code combines the words 'Persia', 'Greece people', 'greater', 'budget', 'Mongolia', 'army'

Option A, 'The Greek army budget is greater than that of Persia or Mongolia' is the correct answer as it uses all the codes, with 'Greece people' being used as 'Greek'.

Question 2

Ω, + 110, ə π, 231, Ƀ

The code combines the words 'army', 'negative employment', 'opposite female', 'Mesopotamia', 'conscription'

Option B, 'Unemployed men are forced to join the Mesopotamia army' is the correct answer as it uses all the codes, with 'negative employment' being used as 'unemployed', 'opposite female' being used as 'male' and 'conscription' being used as 'forced to join'.

Question 3

Σ,(¥ Φ œ), 101 η, Ж, Γ η Z

The code combines the words 'government', 'combine attack greater', 'housing less', 'insurgents', 'terrorists less people'

Option E, 'Terrorist groups and insurgents attacked government house' is the correct answer as it uses all the codes, with 'combine attack greater' being used as 'attacked', 'housing less' being used as 'house' and 'terrorists less people' being used as 'terrorist groups'.

Question 4

η, Ω, Γ , β, T, 999 œ

The code combines the words 'less', 'army', 'terrorists', 'unlawful', 'police', 'weak greater'

Option C, 'Terrorists broke the law and the police were powerless without the army' is the correct answer as it uses all the codes, with 'less' being used as 'without', 'unlawful' being used as 'broke the law', and 'weak greater' being used as 'powerless'.

Question 5

231, Z, χ +, œ + Љ

The code combines the words 'Mesopotamia', 'people', 'health negative', 'greater negative rich'

Option C, 'The population of Mesopotamia suffer from absolute poverty' is the correct answer as it uses all the codes, with 'people' being used as 'population', 'health negative' being used as 'suffer' and 'greater negative rich' being used as 'absolute poverty'.

Question 6

U, η, Σ, κ, 010 œ, 101, 110, (123 312 213 231)

The code combines the words 'budget', 'less', 'government', 'gunpowder', 'policy greater', 'housing', 'employment', 'Mongolia Persia Greece Mesopotamia'

Option D, 'Politically explosive policies on housing and jobs will cut budgets in all countries' is the correct answer as it uses all the codes, with 'less' being used as 'cut', 'government' being used as 'politically', 'gunpowder' being used as 'explosive', 'policy greater' being used as 'policies', 'employment' being used as 'jobs' and 'Mongolia Persia Greece Mesopotamia' being used as 'all countries'.

Question 7

Ω, Ω, 333, Ж œ, δ, λλ, ψ

The code combines the words 'army', 'army', 'inside', 'insurgents greater', 'converse', 'secret', 'meeting'

Option A, 'The army are having a meeting behind closed doors to discuss insurgency within the ranks' is the correct answer as it uses all the codes, with the second 'army' being used as 'ranks', 'inside' being used as 'within', 'insurgents greater' being used as 'insurgency', 'converse' being used as 'discuss' and 'secret' being used as 'behind closed doors'.

Question 8

¥ (Я Z), ψ, ¥ (ə 666), λλ, T

The code combines the words 'combine peace people', 'meeting', 'combine opposite public', 'secret', 'police'

Option E, 'Pacifists meet in private to avoid the secret police', is the correct answer as it uses all the codes. 'Combine peace people' becomes 'pacifists', 'opposite public' becomes 'private'.

Question 9

Options B and C, 'capture' and 'concur', would be the **two** most useful additions to the codes when attempting to convey the message 'Mesopotamia signed a peace treaty with Persia agreeing to release all enemy prisoners.' The word 'concur' being used for 'agreeing' and the word 'capture' being used with the existing code 'opposite' to provide the word 'release'. The other words in the message can be extrapolated from existing codes or are irrelevant.

Question 10

Σ, η, U , Z, χ, γ, Ω

The code combines the words 'government', 'less', 'budget', 'people', 'health', 'comparison', 'army'

Option C, 'The government spending on the army exceeds that spent on citizens' health', is the correct answer as it uses all the codes. The words in the message are paraphrased within the answer.

Question 11

Ω, Σ, 010, 123, ¥ (œ Φ), ¥ (γ Γ̓)

The code combines the words 'army', 'government', 'policy', 'Mongolia', 'combine greater attack', 'combine comparison terrorists'

Option C, 'A military junta is in charge in Mongolia and deals brutally with acts of disaffection', is the correct answer as it uses all the codes. 'Army' becomes 'military', 'government' becomes 'junta', 'policy' becomes 'in charge', 'combine greater attack' becomes 'brutally', 'combine comparison terrorists' becomes 'disaffection'.

Question 12

Persia won the last war with Mongolia and they are now our strong allies.

Option B, '312, =, Ю, 123, ¥ (γ ~), ¥ (ə 999), Э', is the correct answer as it uses the codes required in the statement. The code combines the words 'Persia', 'achieve', 'war', 'Mongolia', 'combine comparison day', 'combine opposite weak', 'allies'. 'Achieve' becomes 'won', 'combine comparison day' becomes 'now', 'combine opposite weak' becomes 'strong'.

Question 13

213, ¥ (γ δ), Ю, 231

The code combines the words 'Greece', 'combine comparison converse', 'war', 'Mesopotamia'

Option D, 'Greece declares war on Mesopotamia', is the correct answer as it encompasses all the codes. 'Combine comparison converse' becomes 'declares'.

Question 14

213, 010, ¥ (η β), β, 101, κ, ¥ (ə E), Ω, Z

The code combines the words 'Greece', 'policy', 'combine less unlawful', 'unlawful', 'housing', 'gunpowder', 'combine opposite include', 'army', 'people'

Option E, 'Greece passed a law forbidding the storage of explosives except by military personnel', is the correct answer as it uses all the codes. 'Policy' becomes 'passed', 'combine less unlawful' becomes 'law', 'unlawful' becomes 'forbidding', 'housing' becomes 'storage', 'gunpowder' becomes 'explosives', 'combine opposite include' becomes 'except', 'army' becomes 'military', 'people' becomes 'personnel'.

Question 15

213, δ, ¥ (ə ~), ¥ (β Z ψ), 333, 213

The code combines the words 'Greece', 'converse', 'combine opposite day', 'combine unlawful people meeting', 'inside', 'Greece'

Option A, 'Greece declares a night-time curfew across the country', is the correct answer as it uses all the codes. 'Converse' becomes 'declares', 'combine opposite day' becomes 'night-time', 'combine unlawful people meeting' becomes 'curfew'.

Question 16

123, 213, 110, Г', ¥ (ə 333 123 213), œ, ¥ (123 213 Ω)

The code combines the words 'Mongolia', 'Greece', 'employment', 'terrorists', 'combine opposite inside Mongolia Greece', 'greater', 'combine Mongolia Greece army'

Option B, 'Mongolia and Greece make use of terrorists from other countries to increase the size of their armies', is the correct answer as it uses all the codes. 'Employment' becomes 'make use of', 'combine opposite inside Mongolia Greece' becomes 'other countries', 'greater' becomes 'increase the size', 'combine Mongolia Greece army' becomes 'their armies'.

Question 17

Persia is demanding that some Greek soldiers face war crime charges.

Option C, '312, ¥ (ə 999 δ), 213, Ω, Z, ¥ (Ю β Φ)', is the correct answer as it is the best way to encode the message 'Persia is demanding that some Greek soldiers face war crime charges'.

The encoding used in the correct answer is 312 ('Persia'), 'combine ə 999 δ' ('opposite, weak, converse') becomes 'is demanding', 213, Ω, Z ('Greece', 'army', 'people') becomes 'some Greek soldiers', Ю, β, Φ ('combine war unlawful attack') becomes 'face war crime charges'.

Question 18

Z, 312, Я , ψ, ¥ (ə η), Φ, γ(Φ T)

The code combines the words 'people', 'Persia', 'peace', 'meeting', 'combine opposite less', 'attack', 'comparison attack police'

Option D, 'People in Persia holding peaceful demonstrations are often fired on by riot police', is the correct answer as it uses all the codes. 'Meeting' becomes 'demonstrations', 'combine opposite less' becomes 'often', 'attack' becomes 'fired on', 'comparison attack police' becomes 'riot police'.

Question 19

¥ (η ~), Ж, κ, 213, Σ, 101, ¥(œ Z), ¥ (œ Φ)

The code combines the words 'combine less day', 'insurgents', 'gunpowder', 'Greece', 'government', 'housing', 'combine greater people', 'combine greater attack'

Option E, 'Yesterday insurgents blew up the Greek parliament building and a large number of people were killed', is correct as it uses all the codes. 'Combine less day' becomes 'yesterday', 'gunpowder' becomes 'blew up', 'government' becomes 'parliament', 'housing' becomes 'building', 'combine greater people' becomes 'large number of people', 'combine greater attack' becomes 'killed'.

Question 20

¥ (+ 123 213 231 312), Φ, ¥ (123 213 231 312), +, =

The code combines the words 'combine negative Mongolia Greece Mesopotamia Persia', 'attack', 'combine Mongolia Greece Mesopotamia Persia', 'negative', 'achieve'

Option E, 'Other countries sometimes invade the Middle East but without success', is correct as it uses all the codes. 'Combine negative Mongolia Greece Mesopotamia Persia' becomes 'other countries', 'attack' becomes 'invade', 'combine Mongolia Greece Mesopotamia Persia' becomes 'Middle East', 'negative achieve' becomes 'without success'.

Question 21

¥ (E Ю), ¥ (œ Z Φ), 213, Ю, 231, π, δ(œ Z)

The code combines the words 'comparison include war', 'combine greater people attack', 'Greece', 'war', 'Mesopotamia', 'female', 'converse greater people'

Option D, 'As with all wars the main casualties when Greece fought Mesopotamia were women and children', is correct as it uses all the codes. 'Comparison include war' becomes 'as with all wars', 'combine greater people attack' becomes 'main casualties', 'war' becomes 'fought', 'female' becomes 'women', 'converse greater people' becomes 'children'.

Question 22

123, λλ, T, γ(Φ Z), ¥ (+ Σ), ¥ (+ =), Ω, Σ, ¥ (γ Φ)

The code combines the words 'Mongolia', 'secret', 'police', 'comparison attack people', 'combine negative government', 'combine negative achieve', 'army', 'government', 'combine comparison attack'

Option A, 'The Mongolian secret police are rounding up dissidents to prevent the military government being overthrown', is correct as it uses all the codes. 'Comparison attack people' becomes 'rounding up', 'combine negative government' becomes 'dissidents', 'combine negative achieve' becomes 'prevent', 'combine comparison attack' becomes 'overthrown'.

Question 23

Options A and D, 'help' and 'protect', would be the two most useful additions to the codes when attempting to convey the message 'To safeguard its borders Greece often came to Mesopotamia's assistance during its wars with Mongolia'. The word 'protect' is used for 'safeguard' and the word 'help' is used for the word 'assistance'. The other words in the message can be extrapolated from existing codes or are irrelevant.

Question 24

¥ (Z 312 Σ), Э, γ(Γ˙ Z), ¥ (123 213 231)

The code combines the words 'combine people Persia government', 'allies', 'comparison terrorists people', 'combine Mongolia Greece Mesopotamia'

Option B, 'Members of the Persian government have close ties with different terrorist groups in other countries', is correct as it uses all the codes. 'Combine people Persia government' becomes 'members of the Persian government', 'allies' becomes 'have close ties', 'comparison terrorists people' becomes 'different terrorist groups', 'combine Mongolia Greece Mesopotamia' becomes 'other countries'.

Question 25

231, Ω, œ, 123, Ω, γ, 312, Ω, +, œ, 213, Ω

The code combines the words 'Mesopotamia', 'army', 'greater', 'Mongolia', 'army', 'comparison', 'Persia', 'army', 'negative', 'greater', 'Greece', 'army'

Options A, 'The Mesopotamian army is bigger than the Mongolian army, comparative to the Persian army, but not as big as the Greek army', and E, 'Greece's army is bigger than those of Mesopotamia, Mongolia or Persia', are both correct as they use all the codes. All of the codes for this message are self-explanatory.

Question 26

¥ (γ Я), ¥ (+ Ю), δ, œ, 213

The code combines the words 'combine comparison peace', 'combine negative war', 'converse', 'greater', ' Greece'

Option C, 'Make love not war was a phrase first used by the ancient Greeks', is correct as it uses all the codes. 'Combine comparison peace' becomes 'make love', 'combine negative war' becomes 'not war', 'converse' becomes 'phrase', 'greater' and 'Greece' becomes 'ancient Greeks'.

Chapter 9
Non-Cognitive Analysis practice subtest

Qu. No	Answer	Qu. No	Answer	Qu. No	Answer	Qu. No	Answer
1	D	26	C	51	B	76	A
2	C	27	B	52	B	77	D
3	B	28	C	53	D	78	B
4	A	29	A	54	B	79	B
5	D	30	B	55	B	80	A
6	B	31	B	56	B	81	B
7	B	32	D	57	A	82	D
8	A	33	A	58	B	83	D
9	A	34	A	59	C	84	B
10	B	35	B	60	B	85	B
11	B	36	C	61	B	86	B
12	B	37	C	62	B	87	B
13	C	38	D	63	A	88	A
14	C	39	A	64	C	89	C
15	B	40	B	65	D	90	B
16	B	41	A	66	A	91	D
17	B	42	A	67	A	92	A
18	B	43	D	68	C	93	B
19	B	44	C	69	A	94	C
20	D	45	B	70	A	95	B
21	C	46	C	71	D	96	B
22	C	47	B	72	C	97	A
23	A	48	B	73	D	98	D
24	A	49	C	74	B	99	B
25	B	50	A	75	A	100	C

101	A	116	D	131	B	146	A
102	B	117	B	132	A	147	B
103	C	118	B	133	A	148	B
104	B	119	B	134	C	149	C
105	B	120	A	135	D	150	D
106	C	121	D	136	C	151	A
107	B	122	A	137	A	152	C
108	B	123	A	138	A	153	B
109	B	124	C	139	C	154	B
110	A	125	C	140	C	155	D
111	B	126	A	141	B	156	1–3
112	C	127	B	142	D	157	3–4
113	B	128	A	143	A	158	4–6
114	B	129	A	144	B	159	4–6
115	D	130	C	145	C	160	1–3

1. Preferred answer: D. Strongly Disagree
   This item measures robustness. Anger and resentment are seen as negative attributes even where there may be some justification.

2. Preferred answer: C. Disagree
   This item measures integrity. You need to be the person that you are and be respected for it. You do not need to pretend to be someone other than you are.

3. Preferred answer: B. Agree
   This item measures empathy. In relation to empathy, this is a measure of sensitivity to others in having the ability to control one's emotions even where provoked.

4. Preferred answer: A. Strongly Agree
   This item measures robustness. A positive answer in respect of individual health would be expected.

5. Preferred answer: D. Strongly Disagree
   This item measures integrity. This is blaming other things for other people's success often irrespective of their actual abilities. It is almost akin to jealousy.

6. Preferred answer: B. Agree
   This item measures empathy. This statement is about having an understanding that there may be reasons or circumstances where people may act out of character and do something bad.

7. Preferred answer: B. Agree

   This item measures robustness. The word 'stress' is often maligned in the workplace, and the individual should be able to cope with the pressures of their work.

8. Preferred answer: A. Strongly Agree

   This item measures integrity. This is a question of honesty, and you should own up to your mistakes.

9. Preferred answer: A. Strongly Agree

   This item measures empathy. An understanding that others may have a tendency to violence, for example, when unable to clearly express themselves, and being in control of one's own anger so as not to retaliate in such situations.

10. Preferred answer: B. Agree

    This item measures robustness. A positive answer would be expected even though circumstances might dictate different strategies.

11. Preferred answer: B. Agree

    This item measures integrity. People have the right to be told the truth, though a degree of sensitivity may be appropriate in the manner they are told.

12. Preferred answer: B. Agree

    This item measures empathy. Showing the capacity to understand another's state of mind or emotion.

13. Preferred answer: C. Disagree

    This item measures robustness. A difficult item to answer that may depend on circumstances, but the item suggests a degree of arrogance and insensitivity therefore the answer would be in the negative.

14. Preferred answer: C. Disagree

    This item measures integrity. This is a difficult item. Although loyalty to an employer is important, there may well be occasions when loyalty to a patient or work colleague is as or even more important.

15. Preferred answer: B. Agree

    This item measures empathy. This statement is about showing sensitivity to a person's behaviour due to circumstances they have found distressing.

16. Preferred answer: B. Agree

    This item measures robustness. This is often a general complaint by employees but a positive response would be expected.

17. Preferred answer: B. Agree

    This item measures integrity. This is about honesty and integrity and admitting when you don't know something.

18. Preferred answer: B. Agree
    This item measures empathy. This measures the capacity to demonstrate your ability to understand and be sensitive with other people.

19. Preferred answer: B. Agree
    This item measures robustness. Being strong-minded or tough-minded would be seen as an advantage.

20. Preferred answer: D. Strongly Disagree
    This item measures integrity. Pretending to be something or someone you are not is a blemish on your integrity.

21. Preferred answer: C. Disagree
    This item measures empathy. This is a difficult item, but empathically it is the ability to understand the other's state of mind and rationalise their reasons and not to retaliate.

22. Preferred answer: C. Disagree
    This item measures robustness. People would be expected to be able to deal with heavy workloads and adopt coping strategies to deal with these.

23. Preferred answer: A. Strongly Agree
    This item measures integrity. Sincerity defines honesty and integrity and thereby is a virtue.

24. Preferred answer: A. Strongly Agree
    This item measures empathy. The ability to be sensitive and intuitive are positive characteristics when dealing with other people.

25. Preferred answer: B. Agree
    This item measures robustness. This is a difficult item to answer and may differ dependent on circumstances. However, generally the answer should be in the affirmative.

26. Preferred answer: C. Disagree
    This item measures integrity. Although these sentiments may be shared by many in respect of some groups of people, the fact remains that all people should be treated equally irrespective of the circumstances; it is important to respect people's rights.

27. Preferred answer: B. Agree
    This may be explained where a person experiences an emotional reaction to the plight of others, e.g. starvation, brutality, natural disasters, and is probably more than just being compassionate.

28. Preferred answer: C. Disagree
    This item measures robustness. This is a difficult item to answer, but on balance the answer should exhibit an ability to undertake a difficult task.

29. Preferred answer: A. Strongly Agree
    This item measures integrity. This is a measure of genuineness that is fundamental to an individual's integrity.

30. Preferred answer: B. Agree

    This item measures empathy. This is the ability to deal with traumatic information in a sensitive way where others may need your understanding to deal with the event.

31. Preferred answer: B. Agree

    This item measures robustness. In medicine it is accepted that patients may have to endure a certain amount of pain during certain procedures, therefore the answer should be positive.

32. Preferred answer: D. Strongly Disagree

    This item measures integrity. It is important to be honest with people, although a degree of sensitivity may be needed on some occasions.

33. Preferred answer: A. Strongly Agree

    This item measures empathy. It is considered important to have the capacity to understand and accept another person's state of mind that may be contrary to your own.

34. Preferred answer: A. Strongly Agree

    This item measures robustness. A positive answer in respect of individual health would be expected.

35. Preferred answer: B. Agree

    This item measures integrity. Frankness and honesty are mutually inclusive, though one can still be sensitive when 'not beating about the bush'.

36. Preferred answer: C. Disagree

    This item measures empathy. Patience is considered an important attribute when dealing with other people who may have difficulty understanding what you're trying to say.

37. Preferred answer: C. Disagree

    This item measures robustness. A difficult item to answer that may depend on circumstances, but the item suggests a degree of arrogance and insensitivity, therefore the answer should be in the negative.

38. Preferred answer: D. Strongly Disagree

    This item measures integrity. This is making judgements about other people who may be in their position as a result of a number of different factors. It does not show respect for others.

39. Preferred answer: A. Strongly Agree

    This item measures empathy. It is imperative that you accept that other people may have very different lifestyles, irrespective of how they may differ from your own morality or personal code of conduct.

40. Preferred answer: B. Agree

    This item measures robustness. A difficult item to answer but, taken at an individual level, i.e. how would you relate the question to yourself, the answer would preferably be in the positive.

41. Preferred answer: A. Strongly Agree

    This item measures integrity. Although there is an element of being judgemental, a position on dishonesty is acceptable and in accordance with the employment of people with integrity.

42. Preferred answer: A. Strongly Agree

    This item measures empathy. It is important to understand and be aware that others may have very different feelings about things than yourself and this always needs to be considered.

43. Preferred answer: D. Strongly Disagree

    This item measures robustness. Anger and resentment are seen as negative attributes, even where there may be some justification.

44. Preferred answer: C. Disagree

    This item measures integrity. People often say this, but the reality is that you are, or should be, the same person with the same integrity at work as you are socially even if your behaviour is more relaxed socially.

45. Preferred answer: B. Agree

    This item measures empathy. This is a measure of the capacity to understand another's state of mind or emotion and is a positive attribute.

46. Preferred answer: C. Disagree

    This item measures robustness. Over-exercising can be indicative of pushing yourself too hard to achieve something, therefore a negative answer would be preferred.

47. Preferred answer: B. Agree

    This item measures integrity. Pretence is not justifiable in any circumstances and honesty is the best policy.

48. Preferred answer: B. Agree

    This item measures empathy. Patience is an important characteristic and demonstrates sensitivity to others even when they may be being difficult.

49. Preferred answer: C. Disagree

    This item measures robustness. This is about pandering to people's egos and such resentment would not be a desirable characteristic.

50. Preferred answer: A. Strongly Agree

    This item measures integrity. This is about being honest and taking all reasonable steps to return something to its rightful owner.

51. Preferred answer: B. Agree

    This item measures empathy. This is the capacity to share and understand another's state of mind or emotion in order to be able to give support to that person.

52. Preferred answer: B. Agree

    This item measures robustness. This is a difficult item for those not used to dealing with others' grief, but the expected answer would be one of being able to detach oneself.

53. Preferred answer: D. Strongly Disagree
    This item measures integrity. Xenophobia is immoral and therefore totally unacceptable.

54. Preferred answer: B. Agree
    This item measures empathy. This is being capable of understanding another person's
    state of mind even when it may differ significantly from your own.

55. Preferred answer: B. Agree
    This item measures robustness. Everyone can have feelings of inadequacy, though
    professionally a person needs confidence in their own abilities.

56. Preferred answer: B. Agree
    This item measures integrity. This is about trust and the expectation that people in
    positions of authority undertake their duties without fear of favour.

57. Preferred answer: A. Strongly Agree
    This item measures empathy. It is a positive attribute to be able to accept and understand
    that other people lead different lives than our own but all should be treated equitably.

58. Preferred answer: B. Agree
    This item measures robustness. When you are speaking to others you often need to be
    sensitive to their feelings and say things in a particular way.

59. Preferred answer: C. Disagree
    This item measures integrity. This says something about the individual and their respect
    for others' position or abilities.

60. Preferred answer: B. Agree
    This item measures empathy. This is the capacity to understand that other people, for
    whatever reason, have some form of addiction and that they need to be sensitively
    handled.

61. Preferred answer: B. Agree
    This item measures robustness. There will often be difficult times at work and you need
    to accept this and carry on.

62. Preferred answer: B. Agree
    This item measures integrity. It is important to be truthful and honest.

63. Preferred answer: A. Strongly Agree
    This item measures empathy. It is a positive attribute to have the capacity to accept and
    understand another's state of mind or emotion, in this case in relation to birth control
    and abortion.

64. Preferred answer: C. Disagree
    This item measures robustness. The characteristics shown socially are the same as those
    shown at work. You need to feel confident in the company of others in order to
    perform effectively.

65. Preferred answer: D. Strongly Disagree

    This item measures integrity. This is a difficult question, and the answer might depend on the circumstances surrounding the mistake. However, generally it is not a useful strategy to always try to blame someone for a mistake that has been made.

66. Preferred answer: A. Strongly Agree

    This item measures empathy. It goes without saying that injured people, irrespective of the circumstances in which the injury occurred, should be treated equally.

67. Preferred answer: A. Strongly Agree

    This item measures robustness. It is often better to defer to others who may have greater knowledge in order to be effective.

68. Preferred answer: C. Disagree

    This item measures integrity. Although it may be accepted that swearing is commonplace in society, that is not a reason or excuse for it to happen in the workplace.

69. Preferred answer: A. Strongly Agree

    This item measures empathy. This is the capacity to accept and understand that mental illness is no different than other forms of illness and work in helping those suffering from it should be fully supported.

70. Preferred answer: A. Strongly Agree

    This item measures robustness. It is important to develop effective coping strategies to deal with the pressures of work.

71. Preferred answer: D. Strongly Disagree

    This item measures integrity. Although dishonesty may be understandable in certain circumstances, it can never be acceptable.

72. Preferred answer: C. Disagree

    This item measures empathy. This is about understanding that others may commit criminal offences but after having served their sentence they have the same rights as anyone else.

73. Preferred answer: D. Strongly Disagree

    This item measures robustness. Anger and resentment are seen as negative attributes, even where there may be some justification.

74. Preferred answer: B. Agree

    This item measures integrity. One is not necessarily a role model as a 'professional' person, but one would expect the integrity of a professional person to be high.

75. Preferred answer: A. Strongly Agree

    This item measures empathy. The capacity to accept, understand and respect that others' beliefs may be different from one's own is important.

76. Preferred answer: A. Strongly Agree

    This item measures robustness. Where people have high expectations of your work it can bring its own pressure and you need to develop strategies to cope with this.

77. Preferred answer: D. Strongly Disagree

    This item measures integrity. There are no degrees of honesty, although there are degrees of how you actually tell someone something, i.e. with sensitivity.

78. Preferred answer: B. Agree

    This item measures empathy. It is always considered better to be a good listener than a good talker. Listening enables you to understand other people and to be more sensitive to their feelings when you do speak.

79. Preferred answer: B. Agree

    This item measures robustness. This is about confidence in yourself and in what you do. We all have things we can improve, but we must learn to like ourselves to function properly.

80. Preferred answer: A. Strongly Agree

    This item measures integrity. It would be expected that your full support would be given to someone with a genuine grievance.

81. Preferred answer: B. Agree

    This item measures empathy. Irrespective of how a person has sustained their injuries, they should be treated as sensitively as any other patient.

82. Preferred answer: D. Strongly Disagree

    This item measures robustness. Running and hiding or burying one's head in the sand is a poor coping mechanism.

83. Preferred answer: D. Strongly Disagree

    This item measures integrity. This is a question about openness and honesty where secrets would not be acceptable. This obviously would not relate to patient confidentiality.

84. Preferred answer: B. Agree

    This item measures empathy. Generally people who give their time to charities are commendable as they are displaying a degree of sensitivity to those who are in need.

85. Preferred answer: B. Agree

    This item measures robustness. Self-esteem is a positive attribute, but going over the top can border on arrogance.

86. Preferred answer: B. Agree

    This item measures integrity. It is an acceptance that there are circumstances, e.g. lifestyle, poverty, where it is understandable why some people are deceitful or dishonest.

87. Preferred answer: B. Agree

    This item measures empathy. This is the capacity to understand another's state of mind and be aware that people may be overwhelmed and reach a breaking point.

88. Preferred answer: A. Strongly Agree

    This item measures robustness. Setting clear goals and often achieving them is the ideal development as long as the goals are relevant.

89. Preferred answer: C. Disagree

    This item measures integrity. This is a difficult item. It really deals with tolerance and the acceptance of others' weaknesses without being too judgemental.

90. Preferred answer: B. Agree

    This item measures empathy. To be sensitive to the problems of the elderly associated with a lack of proper funding is demonstrating empathy.

91. Preferred answer: D. Strongly Disagree

    This item measures robustness. Agitation is the same as anger and resentment and is viewed as being a negative characteristic.

92. Preferred answer: A. Strongly Agree

    This item measures integrity. Integrity is about moral principles and honesty and as such is imperative in professional conduct.

93. Preferred answer: B. Agree

    This item measures empathy. This is the capacity to understand that a person's emotional trauma can be exhibited in different ways that might include hostility and anger.

94. Preferred answer: C. Disagree

    This item measures robustness. This is a difficult item, but at work it sometimes happens that other people need to be confronted and you need to have the skills to do this.

95. Preferred answer: B. Agree

    This item measures integrity. Working within the rules is a necessary and often important part of organisational life.

96. Preferred answer: B. Agree

    This item measures empathy. The capacity to share and understand the feelings of people who are waiting for essential medical treatment is an asset.

97. Preferred answer: A. Strongly Agree

    This item measures robustness. Being able to communicate easily with others and make friends is positive both for work relationships and for giving support in more difficult times.

98. Preferred answer: D. Strongly Disagree

    This item measures integrity. It goes without saying that it is important to always accept responsibility for one's mistakes.

99. Preferred answer: B. Agree

    This item measures empathy. This is about the ability to understand and share another person's feelings. It would seem natural to share and understand that most people would want to die with dignity, even though on occasions this is not possible.

100. Preferred answer: C. Disagree

     This item measures robustness. Being annoyed is the same emotion as anger and resentment and as such is a negative characteristic.

101. Preferred answer: A. Strongly Agree

     This item measures integrity. Being true to yourself is about being honest as to who you are and not pretending to be someone you're not.

102. Preferred answer: B. Agree

     This item measures empathy. This is about the ability to understand and share another person's feelings. Peoples' distress about visiting rules in hospitals is understandable and therefore it is an appropriate reaction.

103. Preferred answer: C. Disagree

     This item measures robustness. A difficult item and circumstances may dictate the answer selected. However, keeping your own counsel can be seen as bottling things up and not coping effectively and therefore a negative characteristic.

104. Preferred answer: B. Agree

     This item measures integrity. The answer to this should be positive in accepting the differences between people, though there may be occasions where the maxim is not appropriate.

105. Preferred answer: B. Agree

     This item measures empathy. Having the capacity to share and understand other people's emotions in bereavement particularly at the time death is pronounced.

106. Preferred answer: C. Disagree

     This item measures robustness. We all want to perform to our best abilities and meet the expectations of others. We will not always be able to do so, but being anxious about it is not effective in promoting confidence and thereby performance.

107. Preferred answer: B. Agree

     This item measures integrity. There is always a possibility that people may be able to tell when you are not being genuine, therefore you should always be who you are.

108. Preferred answer: B. Agree

     This item measures empathy. It is more than likely that other people would be frustrated in these circumstances, and therefore it is an appropriate reaction.

109. Preferred answer: B. Agree

     This item measures robustness. This is a difficult item and borders between high self-esteem and arrogance. A positive view of one's abilities can instill confidence and belief in one's performance, but the slip to arrogance can be very real and problematic.

110. Preferred answer: A. Strongly Agree

     This item measures integrity. You should be the same person, i.e. genuine, whether in the work context or socially.

111. Preferred answer: B. Agree

    This item measures empathy. Sensitivity is an aspect of empathy and therefore family and friends displaying anxiety should be treated sensitively.

112. Preferred answer: C. Disagree

    This item measures robustness. This is a difficult item, and there can be positives either way. However, self-esteem is seen as a successful characteristic in the world of work and it may be better to clearly demonstrate your abilities rather than waiting for opportunities where they may be displayed.

113. Preferred answer: B. Agree

    This item measures integrity. The question may sound sanctimonious but the actuality is that the question relates to your integrity as a person in society.

114. Preferred answer: B. Agree

    This item measures empathy. It should be accepted that everyone at some time experiences the pressure of work and, although we personally may be able to cope with this pressure, there are those who experience significant anxiety and we should accept and be sensitive to this.

115. Preferred answer: D. Strongly Disagree

    This item measures robustness. Anger is a negative characteristic and not conducive to acceptable performance in the workplace.

116. Preferred answer: D. Strongly Disagree

    This item measures integrity. This is a demeaning and judgemental statement suggesting non-professional people have difficulty with what is right and wrong.

117. Preferred answer: B. Agree

    This item measures empathy. This statement is about accepting different lifestyles where people may abuse their health, for example through drug or alcohol abuse, but understanding that they have as much right to receive treatment as anyone else.

118. Preferred answer: B. Agree

    This item measures robustness. Making your point clear is normally seen as being assertive but on occasions may be seen as being argumentative, a negative attribute.

119. Preferred answer: B. Agree

    This item measures integrity. This is about honesty and openness and should be answered in that context.

120. Preferred answer: A. Strongly Agree

    This item measures empathy. This statement is about the capacity to understand another's point of view even when we may fundamentally disagree with it.

121. Preferred answer: D. Strongly Disagree

   This item measures robustness. The answer should exhibit an individual's ability to undertake what might be seen as a difficult task but can sometimes be commonplace.

122. Preferred answer: A. Strongly Agree

   This item measures integrity. It seems obvious that people do want you to be open and honest in what you say but that does not mean being blunt.

123. Preferred answer: A. Strongly Agree

   This item measures empathy. Being calm and friendly can be interpreted as showing understanding and sensitivity and thereby being empathetic when dealing with difficult situations.

124. Preferred answer: C. Disagree

   This item measures robustness. This is a difficult item. People who are more introverted by nature can often be highly skilled in the workplace, but may need to work as part of a team and may have to exert more energy in these situations. However, people more socially bold and extraverted tend to have higher self-esteem and display greater confidence in what they do, which is not to say that extraverts are better than introverts. However, the recognition that personal preferences may need to be put aside when working as part of a team may be required.

125. Preferred answer: C. Disagree

   This item measures integrity. Health and safety rules, irrespective of individual feelings about them, are essentially in place to protect the workforce and their clients.

126. Preferred answer: A. Strongly Agree

   This item measures empathy. This statement is about showing sensitivity, i.e. empathy, to a particularly vulnerable group in society, the elderly.

127. Preferred answer: B. Agree

   This item measures robustness. People who display arrogance about their abilities often alienate others, thereby becoming less effective.

128. Preferred answer: A. Strongly Agree

   This item measures integrity. One would not expect anyone to perform a task other than to the best of their ability.

129. Preferred answer: A. Strongly Agree

   This item measures empathy. Even though you may not have personally experienced the death of a close relative or friend, you should still understand that others have difficulty coming to terms with it even when it is expected.

130. Preferred answer: C. Disagree

   This item measures robustness. It is not considered healthy to take work problems home, and coping strategies should be developed in order to avoid such anxiety.

131. Preferred answer: B. Agree

    This item measures integrity. This shows a degree of conscientiousness in the work an individual performs to make certain they are achieving the required standards.

132. Preferred answer: A. Strongly Agree

    This item measures empathy. This statement is about the capacity to understand another's feelings, in this instance when they are awaiting a serious, even life-threatening operation.

133. Preferred answer: A. Strongly Agree

    This item measures robustness. This is something that most people will have experienced, and it is essential to remain positive in your ability to overcome feelings of self-doubt or self-worth.

134. Preferred answer: C. Disagree

    This item measures integrity. The word 'rebel' almost conjures up someone who is not necessarily trustworthy in respect of how you might expect them to behave. It does not sit well with integrity in a structured environment.

135. Preferred answer: D. Strongly Disagree

    This item measures empathy. Even though you may not have personally experienced bereavement counselling, it is probable that many people benefit from others being empathetic to their situation.

136. Preferred answer: C. Disagree

    This item measures robustness. This is more of an excuse than a reason and shows an element of anxiety in one's own abilities.

137. Preferred answer: A. Strongly Agree

    This item measures integrity. Always aspiring to get things right at work is a basic requirement.

138. Preferred answer: A. Strongly Agree

    This item measures empathy. The statement is about the capacity to accept and understand another's state of mind, in this case not donating a deceased child's organs, even where we may consider this the wrong decision.

139. Preferred answer: C. Disagree

    This item measures robustness. An important coping strategy when feeling low or depressed is to discuss the issues with friends or family. Not letting on is not conducive to workplace performance.

140. Preferred answer: C. Disagree

    This item measures integrity. This is an adage that has probably been around since the beginning of time and tends to promote a blame culture in the workplace.

141. Preferred answer: B. Agree
This item measures empathy. The answer to this statement should be affirmative in that you should have the capacity to accept and understand that people may have strong beliefs that are counter to your own.

142. Preferred answer: D. Strongly Disagree
This item measures robustness. It is important to be positive about yourself, your skills and your abilities. You are unique and the only one who can make things happen is you.

143. Preferred answer: A. Strongly Agree
This item measures integrity. The example is a classic test of a person's honesty.

144. Preferred answer: B. Agree
This item measures empathy. This statement is about accepting that we can all have irrational fears and thoughts and being sensitive to those people that may sometimes be unable to cope with them as well as ourselves.

145. Preferred answer: C. Disagree
This item measures robustness. Having difficulty with people has a negative impact on effective working relationships. Such difficulties need to be confronted with the person or persons concerned.

146. Preferred answer: A. Strongly Agree
This item measures integrity. In acting with integrity a person would in the main adhere to systems and procedures. This does not mean the person would not have the right to question them and recommend change.

147. Preferred answer: B. Agree
This item measures empathy. This statement is a self-assessment of the skills you consider you have that would make you a good counsellor, i.e. empathy, sensitivity and understanding others' state of mind and emotions.

148. Preferred answer: B. Agree
This item measures robustness. High self-esteem helps an individual's confidence without being arrogant and allows others to determine the level of your performance.

149. Preferred answer: C. Disagree
This item measures integrity. There may be one-off occasions where expediency can be used as an excuse to break the rules, but generally this would not be acceptable.

150. Preferred answer: D. Strongly Disagree
This item measures empathy. This statement is giving an either/or scenario whereas all of the attributes, toughness, pragmatism, understanding and sensitivity, are skills that might be appropriate in different situations.

151. Preferred answer: A. Strongly Agree
This item measures integrity. This question concerns 'honesty', and claiming for hours that have not been worked is a clear act of dishonesty.

152. Preferred answer: C. Disagree

    This item measures robustness. This could be described as becoming part of the flock in an effort to gain acceptance even when your values, in this case 'honesty', may be compromised.

153. Preferred answer: B. Agree

    This item measures integrity. In the situation presented, although work colleagues, including friends, appear to have colluded in claiming for hours not worked, it does not mean that you should acquiesce to a 'norm' that is obviously dishonest.

154. Preferred answer: B. Agree

    This item measures empathy. Although claiming for hours that have not been worked is dishonest, it is equally important to empathise with the aggrieved party, in this case your employer, and the loss being caused to their business.

155. Preferred answer: D. Strongly Disagree

    This item measures integrity. Honesty is always the best policy irrespective of the consequences.

156. Preferred answer: 1, 2 or 3

    This item measures integrity. It is being honest in the way that you answer this question. The natural inclination is to answer this positively with a score of 1 to 3, but only you can determine what is the best answer.

157. Preferred answer: 3 or 4

    This item measures integrity. This is a difficult question, and although the preferred answer would normally be in the 4 to 6 range this may not always be appropriate. Certain situations may dictate that you cannot 'be who you are' and the optimum answer would probably be either 3 or 4. This would indicate a degree of flexibility in your approach to situations.

158. Preferred answer: 4, 5 or 6

    This item measures robustness. Irrespective of advice you receive from others, including friends, it is important that you make your own decisions in life and live with the consequences.

159. Preferred answer: 4, 5 or 6

    This item measures empathy. Being able to weigh people up on first meeting them could be described as arrogant. Little is known about that person, their values, opinions, traits, likes, dislikes, etc., and only time will enable you to make a more informed judgement.

160. Preferred answer: 1, 2 or 3

    This item measures integrity. Making an excuse for being late for work or an appointment is obviously 'lying' to avoid any repercussions.